Jake

We cannot [reap?] what we do not [sow] and we cannot sow when we're afraid to plow.

[signature]
10/4/2022

M000205043

TIMED OUT: CHIROPRACTIC

My daughter Tara was a remarkable catalyst for effectively causing life-transforming possibilities all around her. What Tara thought, said and did during her lifetime has affected many lives. For example, she not only saved my life once, but twice. Without Tara, this book could absolutely not be. As you read it, know that Tara is part of your life at this very moment!

This book is dedicated to *Tara Lessard (1972-2019)*

A WORD FROM THOM GELARDI, D.C.
FOUNDER OF SHERMAN COLLEGE OF
CHIROPRACTIC

(SUGGESTIONS AND EDITING BY TONINE GELARDI, D. C.)

It Nettles Men's Minds to Find Truth so Simple! ~Goethe

Philosophy studies the fundamental nature of existence, of man, and of man's relationship to existence. (Philosopher Ayn Rand) The question is not, "Why do you need philosophy?" You have no choice about having a philosophy. Everyone has a philosophy, a set of beliefs, a code of values by which they daily make dozens of big and small decisions. The question is what kind of philosophy you have. It's not about today or tonight; it's about your life. The question is, "Is it carefully decided, objectively based, integrated, and consistent, or is it unconsciously decided, situational, contradictory, opportunistic, and a mishmash of fear-filled beliefs."

In *Timed Out: Chiropractic,* Dr. Claude Lessard clearly articulates and integrates the principles of chiropractic, starting with its major premise. Dr. Lessard helps the reader deepen their knowledge of chiropractic principles and helps them to develop the ability to apply them consistently. Integrity, purpose, efficiency, respect, and success are all greater when we focus on making a life built on consistently sound principles. The author brilliantly develops that the principles of chiropractic are the guidance system (GPS) all chiropractors need to stay focused.

The scientific method can accurately determine an outcome when a single invasive force acts on a static thing. However, as the number of forces increases or that which is being acted upon becomes more dynamic, such as living things, science quickly loses its predictive ability. When substantial numbers of environmental forces act on an extremely complex physical, mental, and spiritual human being, science loses its predictive ability, and we must turn to philosophy, albeit it gives us an imprecise possibility or probability. Science and philosophy are complementary rather than optional sources of knowledge. Both are indispensable in understanding highly complex phenomena, and both are in a never-ending state of improvement.

Professions are defined by their fixed, separate and distinct central area of interest, which is their missions. A central area of interest or mission is a profession's standard of value in areas of research, education, and service activities.

Although D.D. Palmer wrote two books, many journal articles, and gave numerous lectures, I cannot find any evidence that he wrote a formal definition of the profession he founded. The closest thing to a definition I found is the following:

> *Chiropractic is a name I originated to designate the science and art of adjusting vertebrae. It does not relate to the study of etiology or any branch of medicine. Chiropractic includes the science and art of adjusting vertebrae – the know-how and the doing.*
> D. D. Palmer, The Chiropractor's Adjustor, Page 223

There are several descriptions, not definitions, of his profession in his 1910 book, and with minor exceptions, *the one central idea is the adjustment of subluxated vertebrae.*

Philosopher, Ayn Rand, wrote about mission in her famous book, *The Fountainhead*:

> *Nothing can be reasonable or beautiful unless it is made of one central idea, and that idea sets every detail. A building [chiropractic profession] is alive, like a man. Its integrity is to follow its own truth, its one single theme, and to serve its single purpose.* Ayn Rand

Mission drives methods. Several professions that go back thousands of years, whose methods are far from where they started, but their mission has stayed the same. Mission alone identifies every profession. Most people can tell you in a word or two what is central to professions like medicine, obstetrics, dentistry, law, or architecture.

In attending a convention for accredited schools and colleges, a professor offered the following on writing an institutional mission statement. He said:

> *A good mission statement uses action verbs, nouns, and direct objects. It doesn't use many adjectives, adverbs, or passive verbs. Why do some politicians and preachers use many adjectives and adverbs? So that everyone can project their own meaning onto what they say. Everyone can believe that the speaker agrees with their position.*

Which of these mission statements gives you a CLEAR understanding of what their college offers?

1) The mission is to educate and prepare students to become doctors of chiropractic focused on the analysis and adjustment of vertebral subluxation.

2) Chiropractic medicine is a comprehensive health care profession that addresses the wide variety of factors that impact upon human physiology.   Chiropractic physicians specialize in natural, non-invasive health care and are trained to use a full range of medical diagnostic tools and a wide array of effective treatment options in patient care.

The first definition tells what chiropractic is now, will be tomorrow and forever. The mission of the chiropractic profession is to learn more about vertebral subluxation, and to locate, analyze and adjust vertebral subluxations.

The second definition is so broad as to be meaningless. It doesn't distinguish chiropractic from allopathic, osteopathic, or naturopathic medicine. It uses non-invasive methods, but methods do not define professions. Professions are defined by their central area of interest. Those with the same central area of interest are in the same profession. The current non-use of invasive methods is often the result of failed lobbying efforts. Dr. Lessard argues for an emerging new way of seeing with today's knowledge plus a corpus of re-contextualized principles that will inform not just the next generation of chiropractors, but also those they will serve. This book examines these principles with great precision and enthusiasm.

Maintaining health is our preeminent concern because it is the precursor to life abundant.

Hans Rosling, a Swedish professor, found that the data of nations shows that your standard of living "can move up much faster if you are healthy first than if you are wealthy first." (Comparing data on economic prosperity, education, and health, Global Trends TED Talk 2007). The quality of all parts of our life rests on and depends on the foundation of our health.

Health is the high quality of physical, mental, and spiritual life resulting from an innate striving toward active organization, autonomy, and resilience. We try to accumulate constructive health values, recognizing that all processes in nature, both constructive and destructive, take time. Adjusting subluxations removes a major interference to health. Other sources of interference come from lifestyle.

Our bodies tell us what these wrong lifestyle choices are, but we often tell ourselves they are unimportant and won't accumulate. Putting things into our bodies that we know are dangerous sometimes appear enhancing, but the cost to your health often doesn't show up until much later. I believe that many, if not most health problems stem from interferences to health, like vertebral subluxations, and lifestyle. Periodic spinal examinations related to vertebral subluxations are the most effective, safe, and inexpensive part of healthcare that families can engage in.

Chiropractic is an art, as is practiced by all forms of healthcare. Healthcare professions are arts, utilizing philosophy and science. Any professional in music, golf, painting, writing, chiropractic, or other fields work with an economy of motion. They advance their mission with the least intervention. A professional writer can express the most profound emotion with the least number of words. Philosophy influences art: the better our philosophy (and technical skills), the better our art – which is to say that we reach higher levels of professionalism and economy of motion. Our work becomes more specific by advancing our philosophy, art, and science.

Dr. Claude Lessard's *Timed Out: Chiropractic* is an accumulative health value for thousands of patients and doctors. Every chiropractor and every chiropractic student must study this book to enrich their understanding of universal values and of understanding itself.

ENDORSEMENTS

"This was a huge endeavor with countless hours of thoughts, research, investigation and questioning. It is a masterpiece.

A very valuable text for the ongoing evolution, story and saga of chiropractic. It is a milestone document. It will live in posterity. It is not for everyone. It is for the serious intellectual student of chiropractic whether an actual student or a doctor.

I fully endorse it. I am grateful that Claude Lessard, D.C. had the fortitude, foresight, willingness and staying power to produce such a invaluable document."

Arno Burnier, D.C., MLS Seminars, Cafe of Life.

"With his newest book, *Timed Out: Chiropractic*, Dr. Claude Lessard forges new ground in chiropractic thinking. Just when you thought you knew everything about chiropractic philosophy and principles, Dr. Lessard takes you even deeper. Buckle your seatbelt, put on your thinking cap, and keep pressing forward."

Judith Nutz Campanale, DC, ACP- Chair, Board of Trustees Sherman College of Chiropractic

"*Timed Out: Chiropractic,* by Dr. Claude Lessard, is a creative, academic look that weaves Chiropractic's thirty-three principles with current scientific thinking. This journey to the heart of Chiropractic challenges the reader to look through a lens of the 2020's. The book includes new facts and insights on DD and BJ Palmer, reinforcing what the ultimate objective has always been despite having been hidden in marketing and communications. Dr. Lessard uses aviation and computers to help us see how matter is organized and re-organized through a thorough understanding of the basic science of Chiropractic. He reminds the reader that Chiropractic is a philosophy, science and art and that we cannot overemphasize one at the expense of the other two. The basic science of Chiropractic is key to developing the path forward and Chiropractors should enjoy chewing on these deeply important concepts of life, healing and adaptability as they endeavor to bring restoration to the communities where they practice."

William M Decken, DC, FCSC, Chair Philosophy Department Sherman College of Chiropractic

"I took my time so that I could completely digest every word of your newest book. You have created a teaching guide that an individual can use to understand the 33 Principles in their depth, something I've long believed that our profession has needed. This is the perfect compliment to your first book and makes it more understandable. Since most DC's cannot spend a few months in formal study of the foundation of Chiropractic, you have enabled this to become possible without them leaving their office. Thank you for your work and wisdom."

Joe Donofrio, D.C. (Sr)

"The role of innate intelligence is to comprehend universal forces and make them meaningful in the growth and advancement of the living body. Similarly, in the 1920s Stephenson comprehended B.J. Palmer's philosophy and skillfully organized its foundational principles into a systematic framework for the growth and advancement of our profession. Stephenson's Chiropractic Textbook is a testament of the chiropractor's identity in this world; it explains who we are, what we think and how we think.

If words are the scaffolding by which we construct our ideas, Stephenson succeeded in building a framework that remained useful and relevant for decades. Its structure allowed laypeople and scholars alike to understand the big ideas that undergird our profession. Grasping the fundamental concepts in his book is comprehending the unique identity of chiropractic.

The words we use eventually lose their edge and meanings change. In time, ideas need to be explained using newer, more contemporary words. Dr. Claude Lessard has done us the service of re-contextualizing chiropractic's foundational principles with new words: words that are more relevant to this century, words which bootstrap chiropractic foundational principles with ideas to lead us into the next century. Dr. Lessard seeks to bring the chiropractic conversation into the modern age, just as quantum physics will bring society to an all-new level while Newtonian physics remain facts of life. This book helps propel chiropractic forward into a new and exciting future.

Every chiropractor should take the time to understand this book and keep the conversation going."

Joe J. Donofrio DC, ACP, Vice President for Academic Affairs
Sherman College of Chiropractic

"Reading Claude Lessard, D.C.'s Timed Out: Chiropractic was a "welcome home" to me - as it will be for you. He brilliantly upgrades our understanding of Palmer's 33 Principles template, frozen in academic and social models for too long, with a novel exploration of modern wisdom. By helping us to access newer knowledge of self organizing systems, physics, and the linkage of energy and information for manifestation, the 'Big Idea' can now be even bigger for you and those you serve. This is probably the single greatest elucidation of the biggest principles in human history linking historical chiropractic to modern science and expanding the responsibility of the tor to asses for the tic intervention and outcomes that truly represents the real gift for the world. *Warning, this book will crack open your cosmic egg of chiropractic and expand its role in today's world into humanity's next.* **Timed Out: Chiropractic is a foundational must as the basis of our profession and its future. Thank you Claude for your passion and dedication!"**

Donny Epstein, D.C, author, researcher, developer of models of healing, the Network systems for chiropractors, the Energetics **of self organization and creator** *of EpiEnergetics.*

"Claude Lessard, D.C. has an unambiguous understanding of Chiropractic philosophy, science, and art, integrating them in an ardent and engaging way. Using his previous Blue Book, *A New Look At Chiropractic's Basic Science,* as springboard, he unites these three components delving deeply into the thirty-three principles of chiropractic's basic science, demonstrating with accuracy that their instructions are the unequivocal link bridging its philosophy and art. They are, in fact, the GPS system guiding chiropractors to practice the chiropractic objective with singular integrity.

Timed Out: Chiropractic clearly and definitively moves the chiropractic profession into the future.

For the first time, it presents an accurate model of chiropractic based on the indisputable principles of its own basic science!

With a passion we have come to expect, Dr. Lessard clarifies with razor precision, the art of practicing the chiropractic objective applying his new and groundbreaking "hard to vary" universal philosophical explanation."

Tom Gregory, D.C., Certified Spinologist

"As a chiropractic student about to graduate, and I wish I would have had this book in the beginning of school when I first started learning about chiropractic philosophy. Like many of my peers, I had a difficult time understanding Stephenson, mostly because the language he used to describe the 33 Principles was within the context of a different time. In *Timed Out: Chiropractic,* Dr. Claude Lessard redefines the principles with a modern approach that all chiropractors in 2022 could appreciate. D.D., B.J., and Stephenson would be proud of the way that he has expertly bridged the century-long gap between their original theories and today's scientific advancements. Chiropractic is evolving, and Dr. Lessard is at the forefront of this cultural shift. As the new generation of chiropractors, we must be prepared to grow with the profession, and Dr. Lessard is leading the charge!"

Hannah McIntyre, D.C. Graduating Class of Spring 2022

"Timed Out: Chiropractic is a must-read for the Chiropractic Profession. After reading this book it is clear that the 33 Principles are the scientific platform on which the analytical certainty of Advanced Muscle Palpation rests. Chiropractors facilitate and the Innate Law performs the vertebral adjustment! Read this book - and learn from one of the best."

Trent Scheidecker, DC Founder & CEO of ChiroWay & Lead Instructor for Advanced Muscle Palpation

"Occasionally a book is written that brings your mind into new depths and delves into new ways of thinking about time tested principles. It is the rare book and author that can achieve this and get you to question everything you know and bring about new questions. Not only has Dr. Claude Lessard done this once with his book *A New Look at Chiropractic's Basic Science,* but he has gone even deeper into his target the second time with his new book, *Timed Out: Chiropractic.*

I've read this book over and over and each time I find myself being catapulted in my understanding of the science and philosophy of Chiropractic. So many questions have been answered for me in this book, yet I am left with deeper questions to ponder. *Timed Out: Chiropractic* will go down in my humble opinion of one of the great treasures of Chiropractic literature.

There are so many things I love about this book, but I want to share my five top treasures. The first is that I love the brilliance of how Dr. Claude Lessard thinks and the lens in which he presents Chiropractic. Secondly,

I love how Dr. Lessard brings us to the powerful conclusion that what we deemed as our philosophical principles are today's science, which makes the essence of what we do as Chiropractors even more powerful. Third, *Timed Out, Chiropractic* is a book that will get any reader to think and ask questions and want to go deeper into our beautiful profession. The fourth reason I absolutely love this book is because it brings our current understanding of life into time tested principles so that we have a "modernized" version of our principles without interfering with their true meaning. My fifth top reason to love *Timed Out: Chiropractic* is because it literally infused my brain with about 1000 new ways to explain the principles of Chiropractic.

I deeply believe that Dr. Claude Lessard's books should be required reading in our Chiropractic schools. I truly believe that Dr. Lessard is one of the greatest thinkers of our time regarding the 33 principles of Chiropractic. On a personal level being exposed to Dr. Lessard's work has given me a more extensive and powerful understanding of our sacred work as Chiropractors and I am a better human being and Chiropractor because of him and his writings."

Dr. David Serio

FOREWORD

Timed Out: Chiropractic by Dr. Claude Lessard will stretch your mind. The original 33 Principles of Chiropractic, enumerated and described by R. W. Stephenson, were penned in 1927. Stephenson's tome was limited by the vocabulary and technology of the time. His mind conceived concepts for which there were no words. He knew this. In Article 343 of the Senior Text in his *magnum opus* **Chiropractic Textbook**, Stephenson wrote, "We might conceive of this mental impulse as being composed of certain kinds of physical energies, in proper proportions, which will balance other such forces in the Tissue Cell; as electricity, valency, magnetism, cohesion, etc, etc. Perhaps some of these energies are not known to us in physics. What right have we to assume that we have found them all? The writer presents this as a hypostasis or theory in order to get working basis. In other places in this book, other theories for the same thing have been offered, for the same purpose." Tragically, Stephenson died in 1936 and never got to revise his work or see the changes brought about in the later 20th century.

The dynamics of the 20th century brought change that challenged humanity's adaptive capacity: The Great Depression, two world wars, the industrial revolution, and the developments in the fields of transportation, electronics, computers, and space exploration.

I am reminded of an amazing woman, my grandmother, who faced these challenges. "G" as we called her, was born in 1901, shortly after the birth of chiropractic. She saw the transition from horses and dirt roads to automobiles, proudly driving her husband's Essex at a time when women didn't do those things. She refused to fly. Perhaps the safety record of modern jetliners could not supplant her memories of barnstormers, wing-walkers, and the Hindenburg disaster. One of the few times she looked horrified was when she learned I was taking flying lessons.

I remember vividly staying up until the wee hours of the night to watch the first lunar landing on the 21-inch orb of our black-and-white TV. She saw, and participated in, the communications revolution, witnessing the development of the telegraph, telephone, radio, movies, and television. As a young woman, she worked as a telephone operator, and understood wires and switches.

"G" was aware of x-ray, and invited me to watch while an osteopath brought a portable x-ray machine into her bedroom to film a suspected fracture in my aunt. As a child, she and my mother took me to the shoe store where a fluoroscopic examination confirmed the fit. While CT and MRI were developed in her lifetime, I don't think she ever comprehended their significance.

"G" lived to see the most profound changes in science, politics, art, communication, and technology the world has ever seen. Her life was a chronicle of the 20th century. The excitement of seeing transportation evolve from horses to space vehicles, and communication development from the telegraph to the Internet is incomprehensible.

What does all this have to do with chiropractic? Plenty, as chiropractic is the study of life. As exciting as the 20th century may have been, the 21st promises even more dramatic change. Never has the culture been more receptive to our message, and never has the opportunity for personal growth and service to others been greater.

The lessons "G" imparted to her family are values every chiropractor should aspire to: follow your bliss; bring light, love, and encouragement to others; grow with the times; lead and serve by example. My wish is that these principles and values be the legacy of all whose lives we touch, be they family, practice members, colleagues, or friends. I think that covers everyone in the world.

Claude Lessard has taken on the arduous yet joyful task of contemporizing the principles of chiropractic, as our knowledge and vocabulary transitioned from the late 19th century to the 21st century. Precursors to modern quantum mechanics include the 1838 discovery of cathode rays, the 1977 suggestion that that energy systems in a physical system could be discrete, and the 1900 quantum hypothesis of Max Planck. Planck proposed that any energy radiating atomic system can be divided into discrete "energy elements. Each of these energy elements is proportional to the frequency with which each of them individually radiates energy. The 20th century saw the emergence of quantum information science, which crosses disciplines and seeks to understand the analysis, processing, and transmission of information. Quantum theory brought us the mysteries and apparent paradoxes of nonlocality and entanglement.

Lessard first addresses the concept of momentum. In Newtonian physics, momentum is simply mass times velocity. Things get a bit more interesting when we address the momentum of massless particles, such as photons. The velocity of massless particles is an inherent property, And the energy of a massless particle depends on its frequency. As noted in the text, momentum is conserved. While momentum can be transferred from one item to another, the total momentum in the system remains constant. This concept is fundamental to understanding this text.

The bulk of the book is devoted to an analysis and "recontextualization" of Stephenson's 33 Principles, and builds on Lessard's earlier text, *A New*

Look at Chiropractic's Basic Science. The author describes the Guiding Principles (GPS) system for the chiropractic practice objective. The end of the book contains a useful, concise glossary, described as chiropractic's unique glossary.

Lessard describes philosopher of science Karl Popper's assertion that falsification should replace classic inductivist views on the scientific method. The chiropractor is challenged to falsify any of the 33 principles as they are now reclassified.

This book will challenge you. It is not a quick and easy read. It will force you to challenge your premises, biases, and early assumptions. It will guide you through a journey from a 20th-century understanding of the 33 Principles to a new model for the 21st century. Enjoy the journey!

Christopher Kent, D.C., J.D., A.C.P.

references at end of references section

PROLOGUE

READY FOR TAKEOFF

Picture yourself as a passenger on a spacecraft called "Chirotrek", that was launched from Cape Canaveral in July 2017, to get a close look at the planet Jupiter. All you have to do is enjoy the flight and the scenery. Every input to spacecraft Chirotrek will be under the supervision of Houston Control through a complete automated wireless guidance system. They will be using sophisticated software and hardware to keep us on course to Jupiter. Actually, despite the fact that Chirotrek is the size of an average classroom, it is so full of equipment for power generation and space measurements that you and I can't squeeze aboard. But let's imagine.

On the 13th day of our voyage, we accomplish a "space first," videotaping the Earth and Moon together. At day 145, rocket engines get fired briefly from a command of our onboard GPS for a slight correction of our course. At day 210, we cross the orbit of Mars, our nearest planetary neighbor on the voyage to the outer planet.

On day 290, we begin a perilous six month journey through a large band of asteroids, massive tumbling boulders sailing by us ominously as our spacecraft remains on course. Another three months beyond the asteroid belt, we begin to see the massive planet Jupiter clearly, more clearly than any telescope on Earth! It is an immense swirling mass of dense gases and floating clouds, without solid surface or the familiar boundaries between land and sky. Our instruments tell us that the swirling mass is almost completely hydrogen. At its internal center, due to enormous atmospheric pressures, the hydrogen takes on a totally new liquid form called, liquid metallic hydrogen. And now we can also see with precision that outermost room of Jupiter, Callisto, displaying a huge crater from which radiate concentric rings like frozen ripples in a gigantic pond. Next we come to Gaymede, Jupiter's largest moon, with its deeply grooved and mottled icy surface. And then Europa, strangely smooth except for some striations that may be fissures in its thick icy crust. At this point we look for Almathea, and oddly shaped moon, and find in it a ring system that surrounds Jupiter.

Then, on day 600, we are directly adjacent to Jupiter itself, and the famous Red Spot comes into view! We are mesmerized by this giant geyser of complex gases forced from the interior of the planet. But wait, what is this? Yes, a volcano actually in the process of eruption, its bright plume outlined against the darker surface a hundred miles high. Then on day 687, feeling the boost from Jupiter's gravity, control center in Houston resets our course and we are returning back to Earth.

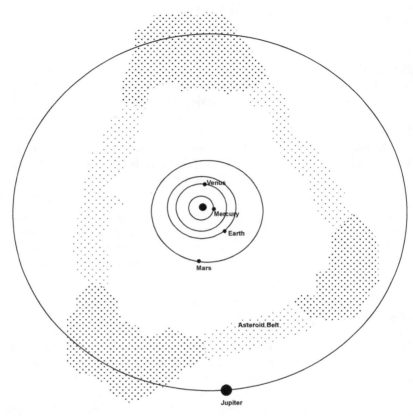

On day 994, we have a brief scare as our GPS malfunctions. We are told by control center that we have lost our fix point as we begin to re-traverse the dense asteroid belt once again. Our spacecraft's optical sensors experienced interference from asteroid dust, altering the momentum of signal transmission. Control center boosted the signal strength, which normalized the transmission of information and guidance was restored. We breathe more easily!

At day 1352, Houston Control transmits signals to our spacecraft's retro rockets to slow us down to about 15,000 miles per hour as we enter our stratosphere. We can now anticipate splash down in the Atlantic Ocean; we are coming to the end of our journey.

Notice that we spent over three and half years on this journey relying on exquisitely intricate aeronautic software of the aerospace industry. Our entire journey was under the direct governance of the control center in

Houston. Employing the most current software, computer hardware, and Guidance Positioning System, control center transmitted information to our spacecraft that kept it on course, and brought us back safely on our beloved planet Earth.

Throughout the text of this book you will find a chiropractic correspondence to the metaphor to "our" space journey.

You will note: the body of a living thing has 100% perfect software that is perfectly updated moment by moment, controlling every computation necessary to adapt to its internal and external environments to keep us on course and alive according to universal laws. Furthermore, as the aeronautic profession continually performs maintenance using pre-check and post-check lists with regularity to insure coordinated systems of connectivity and communication, so is the chiropractic profession performing maintenance using pre-check and post-check lists to insure coordinated systems of connectivity and communication.

Which brings me back to this book of stellar chiropractic connectivity and communication (proving my above narrative), and its re-contextualization filled pages crossing all lines, divisions and boundaries, while remaining on course, as growth and development always do.

As we get inspired as we imagine having been our airspace journey, I assure you that once you've experienced that momentum you'll always want it. So jump on board! We are taking off!

PREFACE

"We never know how far reaching some thing we may think, say or do today will affect the lives of millions tomorrow."

B. J. Palmer, D.C. (1881-1961)

This prophetic epigram underscores the importance of being aware, vigilant, and diligent of the "WHAT" we live for, "WHY" we live in this present moment, and "HOW" we chose to serve.

So, when is tomorrow? Tomorrow starts now in the form of "WHAT" we think, "WHY" we say we say what we think, and "HOW" we live and do what we think. If we need more inspiration, let us consider, together without condemnation, the possibility of seeing something NEW for the first time, that something always before our very own eyes.

The big news? It's plainly about the personal and collective development of our educated intelligence! We could not see what we were not yet capable of seeing. Educated intelligence is the capability of our educated brain to function. It develops and evolves over time, both individually and collectively. The insight of B. J.'s in the quote above could start now for us exactly where we are, and we must take a step forward. We must carry on. The longest journey starts with a single step.

We all have expectations, biases, and personal values. However, there are still universal values that can turn the world upside down. It is always a matter of construction, deconstruction and reconstruction. Chiropractic is at a crossroads at the moment particularly because once again, time is on our side, as we, all of us together without condemnation, grow further into fulfilling our mission of practicing the chiropractic objective exclusively. For that to occur, we need secure and trustworthy guidance, with flawless instructive information and a vigilant system of error correction capable of keeping us on course. This book provides the necessary knowledge to make error correction, so as to become **united** together by the immutable principles of chiropractic's basic science.

This book also points to a NEW evolutionary humanitarian approach to life. It is a re-contextualization of the 33 principles of chiropractic's basic science based on today's knowledge, in 2022, for the student to use alongside Stephenson's textbook. It identifies a huge gap within the practice of chiropractic and firmly closes that gap. It revolutionizes the way chiropractic is constructed and sets it on a solid bedrock platform to be reconstructed upon. It also confronts head on some of the existing practical challenges, from techniques, to research and to intent of purpose for the chiropractor of the future. This book shows how the 33 principles of chiropractic's basic science **unite** chiropractic philosophy and the art of chiropractic practice; how the 33 principles of chiropractic's basic science form a *G*uiding *P*rinciples *S*ystem (GPS) that provides the chiropractor a moment by moment situational awareness for practical correction to keep on course; how the 33 principles of chiropractic's basic science are continually revealing and pointing to the chiropractic objective; and how the 33 principles of chiropractic's basic science can move all of us beyond the confines of our personal values toward the ever expanding universal values of chiropractic itself. So, let tomorrow start right now!

TABLE OF CONTENTS

A NOTE TO THE STUDENT

Consider this work a task book that becomes a NEW chapter in the ongoing story of the continued development of chiropractic that officially began in 1895. The founder, D.D. Palmer died in 1913. The developer, B.J. Palmer died in 1961. The author of "The Chiropractic Textbook", R. W. Stephenson died in 1938. The story of chiropractic has not stood still since. We **carry on** and build on the knowledge that we inherited from these giants. We are also moving forward, always reaching for a deeper and greater understanding of chiropractic. This book has its own pre-requisites. First, every section of Stephenson's 1927 textbook should be studied completely. Even within the context of its time, with its theistic and anthropomorphic assumptions, it is a most comprehensive and necessary introduction to chiropractic. The information it contains is extremely valuable as it provides the foundational background most needed to understand the breath and depth of the chiropractic body of knowledge as it continually unfolds. It is important to know that Dr. Stephenson's textbook was fully approved by Dr. B.J. Palmer, who exalted Stephenson and his book in this letter of approval,

DOCTOR PALMER'S LETTER OF APPROVAL OF CHIROPRACTIC TEXT BOOK

Dear "Stevie":

I could not blame you if you have grown impatient at my apparent silence in not giving you an expression of my opinion regarding your MSS. which you submitted for my approval or disapproval.

I have been doing some writing, taking my time to think it over carefully; and, between times when tired, I would go over another chapter of your book.

This is Sunday and I have just finished it. Of ALL the books written and compiled on Chiropractic Philosophy, this is by far the best, not excepting my own. The one great, grand and glorious thing you HAVE done has been to compile the many principles which are in my writings, into a systematic, organized manner, building them up from simple to the higher forms, so that any layman inclined could investigate and find out what CHIROPRACTIC IS, IS NOT; WHAT IT DOES AND DOES NOT; HOW AND WHY IT DOES WHAT IT DOES. YOU have clearly, carefully and consistently compiled the many PRINCIPLES of Chiropractic into a readable, understandable book, simple enuf for the layman, deep enuf for the savant.

My writings are many. They are in one form or another; either here or there. Each subject is exhaustive. If any person wanted full and complete information on a specific subject, then vii LETTER OF APPROVAL he should go to the special monograph on that subject, but, if he wants the working approximate principle then in your book he gets them all.

Where has always been a void in Chiropractic literature. Assuming an understanding mind asks where he can get a book which would tell him what Chiropractic is—I have always felt that there was no one specific work that we could hand him for that purpose. WE NOW HAVE THAT BOOK. It is your work. You have filled a niche that no other work has done. Here is a book that any chiropractor can hand to any investigating lay mind and know that it will do him, Chiropractic and yourself justice. Your work can now be used as a handbook on that subject.

I rejoice with you in its production.
              As ever,
              B. J. "[1: p. vii-viii]

Second, the book entitled "A New Look At Chiropractic's Basic Science" is a must and should be read with a beginner's mind (one who chooses to continuously be welcoming NEW possibilities) as it leads to a greater understanding of the ever-growing development of chiropractic. It is B.J. Palmer, in 1934, who wrote,

"IN ENTERING into the study of this book and its work, each should, so far as possible, lay aside for the time being all previous theories, beliefs, teachings, and practices. By so doing, you will be saved the trouble of trying, all the way thru, to force "new wine into old bottles." If there is anything, as we proceed which you do not understand or agree with, let it lie passively in your mind until you have studied and gone thru the book the THIRD time, for many statements that would at first arouse antagonism and discussion will be clear and easily accepted further on, after mature reflection and after repeated understanding. After you have given the book mature deliberation, if you wish to return to your old beliefs and ways of living, you are at perfect liberty to do so. But, for the time being, become as little children; for said the Master, "Except ye become as little children, ye can in no wise enter the kingdom of heaven "[2: p. copyright]

I must point out that we are indebted to our predecessors in a monumental way. It so happens that the book, that you are about to study, is facilitated by the 33, already discovered, principles of chiropractic's basic science that are being used to verify its content. Therefore, every thought developed throughout this book reflects the actual guidance of the 33 principles to make the necessary error corrections for chiropractic to continuously move forward, only if it is possible, according to universal laws (pri. 24).

N.B. Throughout the book I have capitalized some of the text to emphasize the importance of the content expressed. Much of the emphasis consists of NEW information that needs NEW receptive educated brains in order to continually grow chiropractic into its promising future.

HISTORICAL BACKGROUND

At the very beginning of the Senior Text Stephenson wrote,

"Art. 304 DATES.

The history of Chiropractic is really the history of adjustments."
Quotation from Volume IV:

*"Although Chiropractic was not so named until 1896, yet the naming of 'Chiropractic' was much like the naming of a baby; it was nine months old before it was named. Chiropractic, in the beginning of the thoughts upon which it was named, dates back at least five years previous to 1895. During those five years, as I review many of these writings, I find they talk about various phases of that which now constitutes some of the phases of our present day philosophy, showing that my father was thinking along and towards those lines which eventually, suddenly crystallized in the **accidental** case of Harvey Lillard, after which it sprung suddenly into fire and produced the white hot blaze." (B. J. Palmer)*

As Chiropractic grew, other important things useful in Chiropractic were discovered: Palpation, between 1898 and 1900; Nerve Tracing, 1905; Meric System, 1909; Spinograph, 1910, Taut and Tender Fibers, 1922; Neurocalometer, 1924. (Note I heard B. J. explain Taut Fibers in 1920 in his classes, as if it were then old to him. But no one seemed to pay much attention to it until in 1922, when he began to emphasize it; so, 1922 is the date usually mentioned. R. W. S.) "[1:p.230]

For a brief history, I will quote Stephenson's textbook:

"Art. 305 HISTORY OF ADJUSTING.

"I prefer to quote B.J. Palmer in 'Majors and Minors,' p.7, in order to tell the History of Adjustments:

*"The first patient who received a Chiropractic adjustment was Harvey Lillard, a colored man. The **incident**, in brief, follows. He had been deaf 17 years, so much so that from the Fourth Floor of the building where he was janitor he could not hear wagons moving or streetcars rolling on the streets below. When asked how he became deaf, his explanation follows: 'While, in a cramped, stooped position, I felt and heard something pop in my back. Immediately, I went deaf.' To one who was observant, a student, that would be an accidental eye-opener, and it was D.D. Palmer who asked, 'What is the connection between the back and hearing in the ears?' He examined the back.*

By good fortune, the first case in which a spine was examined with that thought in view, a LARGE bump was found. It was not one of the common bumps we see today in palpation, but so prominent it could be seen with the eye.

The following consequential reasoning occurred. If there was no bump when the hearing was good, and the production of this bump destroyed hearing, why don't the reduction of the bump restore hearing? The first attempt to correct what is now a subluxation, was then made. The patient was put upon the floor, face down, and a shove-like movement given. The "bump" was reduced by the first three shoves, and in three days hearing was restored. Harvey could hear a watch tick at the average distance you and I can today.

"The next question was, if the reduction of one bump in one man restores hearing, why won't a similar bump, in other people, produce deafness, and if it does, why wouldn't the reduction of these bumps, in the same way, restore their hearing? It was tried on others. By a peculiar series of circumstances, the results did not come as readily in their cases, but eventually they came.

"Then the third question arose: If a bump in the back caused deafness, why not other parts of the spine produce other dis-ease? So our question has gradually enlarged until by a systematic systemic series of investigations, covering years, you have your Chiropractic of today.

"Education advanced. After a period we ceased calling them 'bumps.' They became 'dislocations.' We, at a later time, were impressed with the idea that this bump was not a dislocation. It was, in reality, not a dislocation but partial, more assuming the character of a luxation, yet not a luxation. It was a subluxation.

"When we had assumed, as a matter of education, that breadth of ideals where they became subluxations, we no longer assumed to shove. We developed the 'push and pull principle,' which was of various forms and methods.

"We began, at a following period, to study the spine from a MECHANICAL point of view. Until this time the only people who attempted to study the spine, as a machine, were osteopaths, although pathologically they still regarded man as chemistry and physics.

"We confined our observations of mechanical ideas to the spine, so much so that we brought out the 'Knowledge of the Kinematics of the Spine'; both normal and abnormal, as to position, apposition, and *subluxations. We then began the study of the pathological, traumatic and anomalous conditions of the spine. At that time began the gathering of the osteological collection which we now possess, for the purpose of elucidating the theories then held and propagation of others.*

"It became necessary that we know the human spine. That was the keynote of the study of CAUSES of diseases of man. We studied spines of all characters; thousands of other bones that we might better reach a new thought or idea in progress. How well that has been done you know today. Hours, months, and years were spent in the study of 'dead bones' to be able to give thoughts that may be taught in a few minutes. Yet it took years to reach the conclusions given in a few minutes.

"When we studied the spine, mechanically speaking, we realized that 'treatment' was far-fetched in its application, as describing the thing we attempted to do. Being a machine, mechanically constructed, mechanically subluxated, it should be mechanically ADJUSTED. Then came the word 'adjustment.'

"Approximately six years ago we began a series of clinical tests or investigations from a new viewpoint. I refer to the Spinograph. Until that period the X-Ray had not been used in its application to human spines in living individuals for the purpose of ascertaining the approximate detailed apposition of the vertebrae, normal, abnormal and traumatic. When we made our first series of Spinographs we were the first to touch this vital question. There existed no previous technique for our observations or work. It became necessary to develop a system of taking spinographs to prove that subluxations existed, where and of what character.

"We began tabulating these observations, which today we are ready to say makes another step. These conclusions are based on the readings and studies of over 50,000 spinographs, all of which were taken in our laboratory with this definite end in view.

"It is no longer sufficient to say that we adjust with the recoil. We are ready for our next step, which you may call '206,' altho I prefer the 'Toggle-Recoil' because of its application by the new series of observations made from the spinographic facts.

"History is 'his-story.' The 'his' in this case being the author who has lived it, been the cause for a large majority of it, therefore the source of the facts here recorded could not be improved." (B. J. Palmer)
[1:p. 230-233]

Some 12 years later, it is August Dye D.C., in "THE EVOLUTION OF CHIROPRACTIC" who wrote,

> *"The history of Chiropractic begins with its **"accidental"** discovery by D. D. in 1895. The evolution of Chiropractic really begins with the departure of the Founder from active teaching of his discovery and his leaving the management of affairs in early Chiropractic history to his son, in 1902. "*[3: p.12]

I mentioned August Dye to verify and confirm that it was an **"accidental"** discovery. B.J., Stephenson and Dye, agree about how D.D. Palmer came to discover this NEW way of understanding the human body. Dye went on to describe "his-story" when he wrote,

> *"Linked with the name of the Discoverer and Founder of Chiropractic is that of its first patient. That patient was Harvey Lilliard, the negro janitor of the Putnam Building in which D. D. had his office. That was a small Office, divided into two rooms, one of which D. D. called his Treatment Room, the other his Reception Room and private office. Harvey was so deaf that he could not hear the noises of the horse-drawn traffic on the street four floors below, nor could he hear the rumbling of the trolley as it rounded the corner. Being interested in the welfare of the sick, as a practicing healer and as a student in search of a means to more effectively treat the sick, D. D. was naturally interested in Harvey's case.*

> *Just how D. D. noticed the spot on the back of Harvey's neck, which he thought might have some relation to the cause of his deafness, there is no recorded history other than as I shall relate it here,—an **incident** every Palmer graduate and student has heard from the lecture platform or read in articles on early Chiropractic. I mean the exact circumstance that induced D. D. to look to Harvey's spine in the first instance. The deductions leading D. D. to do this are doubtless pasted in B. J.'s Scrap Book, in the Founder's notes made at the time. All that is now definitely known is that D. D. discovered it as a part of his investigation. I have heard B. J. relate the incident in many a lecture before the student body at the P. S. C., and D. D. himself has described it to me in very much the same manner as B. J. tells it.*

> *One day when Harvey was doing his work, the Founder asked him, "How long have you been deaf, Harvey?"*

> *Harvey answered him, "Over seventeen years, Dr. D. D."*

D. D. then asked, "How did it happen? What brought it on, Harvey? Do you know?"

Harvey answered that one day as he was bent down in a stooped position doing his work, all at once he heard something pop in his back, and he became deaf almost immediately after and had been deaf ever since. D. D. asked if his back had hurt him at the time he heard this popping, and if it still hurt him. Harvey said that it did hurt him at the time, that he still had pain there.

D. D. then asked Harvey if he could see his back, thinking perhaps he could find something there to give him a clue as to the cause. Harvey removed his clothing so D. D. could examine his back, to see if he could find this clue or any evidences remaining of the location of that popping sound and the pain Harvey noticed at the time he became deaf and which pain he still had.

D. D. examined Harvey's spine. In so doing he discovered an unusually large lump or bump at the back of the neck, at the region since determined to have been the fourth cervical vertebra. He examined all about the place, pressing about it and on it, much as the Chiropractor does perhaps in making a nerve tracing today. While doing so he asked, "Does that hurt, Harvey?"

Harvey said, "Yes, doctor, that is sore all of the time."

D. D. then asked, "Is that where you felt sore right after you heard this popping sound?"

Harvey answered that it was, and that it had been more or less tender ever since. D. D. asked if he might "treat" that bump, to which Harvey assented. Following this, in a fashion that in the light of later developments in Chiropractic adjustic technique must be considered crude, the first adjustment was given. D. D. had Harvey to lie down on the floor, face downward, and he gave the first Chiropractic patient a poke or a push in the neck to see if he could reduce that bump and perhaps help Harvey rid himself of the deafness.

Lo and behold! Following this adjustment—for adjustment it must be considered, no matter how crudely done—when that lump was given a push or a shove by D. D. the deaf man was almost instantly enabled to hear the noises of traffic in the streets below and to hear D. D.'s voice spoken in a normal tone, something he had not been able to do for over seventeen years. After repeated "treatments" for several succeeding days, Harvey Lilliard was as able to hear as any other person possessed of normal hearing. For several years thereafter he worked at his trade about town, his last employment having been as janitor as the Davenport City Hall.

From its discovery made in that homely, crude fashion, in the simple adjustment of a lump discovered at the back of the neck of this lowly workman, on that date memorable in Chiropractic's history— September 18, 1895,—dates the beginning of the evolution of the Art, Science and Philosophy of Chiropractic. Along with its Discoverer and Founder, the name of Harvey Lilliard, a humble, lowly janitor, is revered by all who have a love of the Chiropractic principle for the benefits it has conferred on humanity.

D. D., following his success in this, his first Chiropractic patient, continued his experimenting and adjusting of bumps and lumps at the backs of the necks of those of his patients who would submit to the torturous thrusts and pokes then given by him. He was remarkably successful from the very start in this new form of hand treatments, as D. D. called his early adjustments "[3: p.12, 31-32]

QUANTIFYING THE KNOWLEDGE
OF THE TIME

B.J. mentioned above, "that education advanced." It is true that educated intelligence, which is the capability of the educated brain to function, continually grows over time, individually AND collectively, from generation to generation. Human beings are not born fully equipped with levels of morality, values or physical prowess. They come to those levels after several major stages of development. We easily observe this truth in an infant. At birth, the educated brain of a newborn does not have much capability to function since it does not have many experiences and understandings, therefore its educated intelligence is rather undeveloped. As its educated brain grows so does its capability to function. For example, take a child age 3, and show her a ball that is colored half red on one side and half orange on the other side. Show her red and say "red". Show her the color orange and say "orange". Then show her the color red and ask her what color she sees and she says "red". Show her orange and she says "orange." Now, sit on the floor with her sitting in front of you. Put the ball between both you, with the red side of the ball facing her, then, ask her, "What color do YOU see?" The child is all excited and says, "Red." Then ask her, "What color do I see?" And she will say, "Red". The child cannot take your point of view as she is thinking that what she is seeing is exactly what you are seeing, also. She is not trying to be contrarian, disrespectful or obnoxious, she just does not have the capability to see you as an individual separate from her. However, wait until the child is 7 years old, and repeat this experiment. Then ask the child what color she is seeing and she will say "Red" and ask her, "What color do I see," and she will say, "Orange." What happened between age 3 and age 7? The capability of her educated brain has grown to be able to include your point of view into her life. Her educated intelligence has developed to a point to be able to accept you as being different than her. There is a differentiation that occurred over time between her perceptions of you as an, "other" person. At 3 years old, she could not really see you as you. She only saw you as herself. It was not due to a repression on her part. It was simply that her educated intelligence had not yet developed to be able to do this at all, and so the child lacked it. It was not her fault, as she was not repressed. It simply was that the capability of her educated brain had not grown to be able to "see" the reality of differentiation yet. This lack is not due to repression, but to lack of development.

In 1895, the "*ACCIDENTAL* eye-opener" did occur pretty much in the same way. D.D. Palmer saw exactly according to the capability of his educated brain to function at the time he observed his janitor's back. He saw a LARGE "bump" protruding from the spine and pushed on it several times. That's what D.D. observed. That's HOW, according to D.D., the hearing of Harvey Lillard was restored. D.D. reasoned according to the capability of his educated brain to function, *within the CONTEXT of 1895*. He actually THOUGHT he had found the cure for deafness and eventually of all diseases. This is how D.D. Palmer began to promote the idea of "getting sick people well" by examining the spine and pushing on the bumps he could see. It was not D.D. Palmer's fault that he could only rationalize within the therapeutic model of "getting sick people well." D.D. could NOT reason any differently than what he COULD reason. He simply reasoned according to the development of his educated intelligence and with his accumulated knowledge of the 1890's. Using rational logic, D.D. knew that he had discovered something NEW that was not medicine or surgery. He then set out to construct the SCIENCE, ART and PHILOSOPHY of chiropractic based on his educated intelligence, and the context of his day to get sick people well by attempting to cure their ailments through his *"hand treatments."* D.D. wrote, "I systematized and correlated these principles, made them practical. By so doing I created, brought into existence, originated a science, which I named Chiropractic; therefore I am a scientist"[4: p.818]. He also mentioned that he answered the question, "What is life" and said, "Therefore I am a philosopher." It is clear that D.D. was a pioneer who had a great affinity for wanting to help the sick get well. He was already a magnetic healer. He had a sizable practice at the time. He discovered chiropractic and set out to construct its science, its art and its philosophy. He also claimed, early on, that chiropractic could "get sick people well" better than medicine, and that, without drugs and surgery! This is what Stephenson wrote about the three aspects of chiropractic, "Put simply, that means, 'what it is, how it is done, and why.' SCIENCE tells us what it is; ART tells us how it is done, and PHILOSOPHY, the 'why' of the other two"[1: p.xiv]

At the very onset, chiropractic was used as a therapeutic way of "getting sick people well." In the early phases of chiropractic, relieving the sufferings of humanity was WHAT the chiropractors thought chiropractic's primary goal really was. We must remember, that in the 1890s, the principles had not been formulated yet. For chiropractors then, it meant to provide a service that was superior to medicine in order to "get sick people well." The majority of the early students of D.D. Palmer were medical doctors. Chiropractic philosophy was about understanding the relationship between the non-material and the material. There was a certain advantage, for these early students, to be using chiropractic as an "add-on" to their treatment procedures to get sick people well some of the time. D.D. could not have foreseen that the chiropractic objective would eventually be revealed, through the 33 principles of its basic science, as **EXCLUSIVELY** being the correction of subluxations for the restoration of **transmission** of innate impulses, nothing else. The educated intelligence of D.D. Palmer was still growing and developing further in thoughts those early days; he eventually saw that, "Chiropractic is manual --- done by the hand, but it is not therapeutical, does not use remedies"[4: p.397] What D.D. eventually realized around 1906, was that "The principles of Chiropractic should be known and utilized in the growth of the infant and continue as a safeguard throughout life".[4: p.56] D.D. seemed to be moving away from "getting sick people well"; however by that time, D.D had already taught chiropractic to his early students who were then teaching it to others. This is how chiropractic had its beginnings that were misconstrued, taking a direction of personal views, and started to divide into factions as an early profession. The universal values of chiropractic were being deformed, by these early students, and reformed into their own personal values, that were excluding people without medical conditions. In the words of D.D., "... there is one thing I note, that when I teach the science to one person and that person teaches it to another and the third person teach it to the fourth, that they get away from the chiropractic until in the hands of the third or fourth person is hardly recognizable as chiropractic".[5: p.27-34] Thus the prevalence of "getting sick people well" completely engulfed the minds of the majority of chiropractors all over. Chiropractic has been practiced well before it was understood for WHAT its objective really is. Hence, it was with a constant struggle and disagreements, at the early beginnings of a young profession, that the first chapters of the story of chiropractic were being written. May the NEW chapters of this magnanimous story, continue to be written for posterity, at least, for the next 5000 years!

MOVING FORWARD (2ND CENTURY)

"In Science, the thing is to modify and change ones ideas as science advances."   Claude Bernard

This quote of Claude Bernard signals the necessity for the application of the principles of a science of any profession that we should constantly look for errors and make appropriate corrections.

In the second century of chiropractic, we acknowledge that the universal values of chiropractic are revealed through the 33 principles of its basic science. We acknowledge that chiropractic gets "sick people well" SOME of the time, and fails some of the time. We also note that "getting sick people well" is **"ACCIDENTAL"** to chiropractic care. We understand that any method of "getting sick people well" has its successes and failures. However, we must remember that the 33 principles of chiropractic's basic science are "of a CAUSE and not effects".[1: p.93] It's never too late to make error correction and get back on course! It is worth repeating, D.D. died in 1913. R.W.S. died in 1938. B.J. died in 1961. The world of chiropractic has not stood still since. We have built on the knowledge that we inherited from these giants, but we are also moving on. After all, D.D., B.J., and R.W.S would certainly want us to **CARRY ON** their work, just like Reggie Gold charged us to **"CARRY ON"** the week before he died in 2012.[6]

It must be pointed out that this **"ACCIDENTAL"** discovery, of conduction of information/forces, was a collective discovery due to the collective development of educated intelligence found in other fields of endeavor. Edison, Marconi, Bell, Morse and Palmer (from 1850 to1900) were all discovering the principles of conductivity within their respective fields. Why? Because, educated intelligence grows collectively, as well as individually within the CONTEXT of every era. (For example, classical music: Bach, Mozart, Beethoven, Brahms in the 1700s, --- quantum physics: Maxwell, Einstein, Bohr, early 1900s, --- the computer: AlanTuring, John von Newman, Douglas Hartree in the1940s, --- new chiropractic schools: Sherman College, Life University, ADIO Institute, Spinology, 1973-1980, --- the internet: Bill Gates, Steve Job, Mark Zuckerberg, in the 1980s, etc...). It reinforces the fact that ALL of us are truly influenced according to the development of our own educated intelligence. The individual mind is really a prisoner of its time and simultaneously enticed to go further.

Today, with additional discoveries and new knowledge, we are ALL positioned to **CARRY ON** and further the work of our predecessors. Chiropractic has continually evolved as education advanced.[1: p.232] Our understanding of chiropractic is constantly growing as well. This book will point to the fact that as early as the 1920's, chiropractic's basic science describes the very nature of chiropractic (the WHAT chiropractic IS). When *The Chiropractic Text Book* was first published in 1927, it was crystal clear that chiropractic is about correction of subluxations for the restoration of the **transmission** of innate (mental) impulses that is the link of the relationship between the three united factors of the "Triune of life" (universal life, i.e., existence) and nothing else.[1: p.270] Then why did we miss it? Because, as we mentioned earlier, the capability of our educated brain had not developed as it is today. We must not forget that the prevailing conception of that time was "to get sick people well" without drugs or surgery, and that many of the first chiropractic students were medical doctors. Chiropractic was thought to be the cure of diseases, and could do it better than medicine.

The 33 principles of chiropractic's basic science reveal that there can be interference with transmission of innate information/forces (pri. 29) caused by vertebral subluxations (pri. 31) and that interference violates the principle of coordination (pri. 32). Therefore, the chiropractic objective has always been the location, analysis and facilitation of the correction of vertebral subluxation for a normal transmission of the conducted innate information/forces. PERIOD. It was the chiropractors, themselves, WHO chose to use chiropractic for their own personal agendas that focused on the limited possibility of "getting sick people well" some of the time. That was their surmising from 1895, and it has been carried all the way up to now. Yet, chiropractic's basic science is comprised of principles that are based on *what is possible ALL of the time*. Chiropractic's humanitarian and evolutionary approach constantly needs adjustments, for error correction, to stay " on course" or "in flow", to follow the trajectory and the unfolding of chiropractic's future. This task book is a NEW chapter to help **CARRY ON** the narrative that our predecessors began in 1895. We owe them so much.

CLARIFICATION

Over the years, skeptics have asked whether chiropractic was a science. To them, chiropractic looks not like a science but a set of beliefs and philosophical concepts about them. Skeptics are not to blame, as we read in the background above; chiropractic was **"accidental"** and quite intriguing due to being a NEW discovery (i.e. never before observed.) It is worth verifying that chiropractic is really a science, as well as an art, and a philosophy. Therefore, a framework inspired by science is useful and meaningful. To be accepted as a science, chiropractic must satisfy some criteria:

1. A systematically organized body of knowledge: chiropractic is 33 principles concluding to an absolute irrefutable objective.

2. An experimental method: applying the 33 principles to practice the chiropractic objective through the location, analysis, and facilitation of the correction of vertebral subluxation.

3. Reproducibility: of the locating, analyzing and facilitating the correction of vertebral subluxations through pre and post checks.

4. Testable, verifiable, or falsifiable hypotheses through the chiropractic objective concluded from the 33 principles.

5. Specific predictions from chiropractic applied science to achieve the chiropractic objective. The application of the principles of chiropractic's basic science is for living things, more specifically the living vertebrate body.

6. Natural things as cells, organs, functional systems, and living bodies that provide a sequence of representations, in which each transmission of conducted information/F for coordination of activities is under an innate control to demonstrate the absolute necessity of correcting interference in transmission (vertebral subluxation).

In my book, *A New Look at Chiropractic's Basic Science*, those criteria were analyzed and it was concluded that chiropractic's basic science met them all. It was also clarified that energy and matter are comprised of the same subatomic particles (electrons, neutrons and protons) with different configuration and velocities, making them interchangeable.[7: p.59] This means that energy and matter are one and the same. Therefore, "force" in chiropractic, which is the second factor of the Triune of Life (pri. 4), cannot be energy since energy is the mass of matter at the square of the speed of light ($E=mc^2$). Energy and matter are interchangeable.

Force, in chiropractic, is **information**. Information is non-discrete (can not be divided into parts). Stephenson did intuit about it when he wrote, "General Sense is information which Innate receives."[1: p.178]

However, he never expounded the concept any further. This clarification has been demonstrated at my 2019 Sherman College IRAPS keynote presentation. (Throughout this book I will refer to Energy/matter as *"E/matter"* and to information/force as *"information/F"*).

In some respects, information/F is an abstraction of a particular principle, be it of an organized interstellar galaxy, of an organized universal computer, or of an organized body of a living thing. Information/F is organized in symbols in the form of codes in order to communicate a message. The innate law of the human body has always controlled and organized information/F, for use in every cell of the body, through adaptation, computation, and encoding (pri. 20, 23). Then from this encoding information/F it constructs new cells through its own computational methods.

That is precisely WHAT the 33 principles of chiropractic's basic science are all about. These 33 principles are congruent with all of the laws of conservation, and they explain some aspect of the laws of motion as consequences of a universal regularity in nature. The chiropractic objective concluded from those 33 principles is to locate, analyze and facilitate the correction of vertebral subluxation for a normal transmission of conducted innate information/F of the body. PERIOD.

As an analogy, it is for a receptor (receiving tissue cell) to receive a message from a CPU computer (brain cell) through a medium, which is a transmitter (nerve cell). It explains that the receptor, computer, and transmitter are physical systems. Stephenson wrote, "This might be called the Physical Triunity. It is the physical representation of "Brain Cell" and "Tissue Cell" and the "Link" between them, as spoken in the Freshman work."[1: p.164] However, note that the message is not physical. It is information/F, initially organized and assembled, then encoded as instructions in the computer. It is then propelled through the transmitter and decoded by the receptor. The overall process constitutes, to the observer, **what is possible** in terms of adaptation and computation; it also points to a possibility of interference of the transmitting nerve (pri. 29). This interference, the subluxation, would alter the momentum of flow of the innate impulse (pri. 31), thus altering the timing of the encoded data necessary for normal transmission of the message, and violating the principle of coordination (pri. 32).

I will draw on several disciplines of science to demonstrate that chiropractic's sciences (basic and applied) **unite** chiropractic philosophy and chiropractic art. I will also point to the fact that in chiropractic, the philosophy, the science, and the art, each retain their respective identity as being separate and distinct from each other. It is ONLY through the integration of those three aspects of chiropractic that the chiropractor can choose to practice the chiropractic objective, and EXCLUSIVELY the chiropractic objective.

The intent of this book is to write a NEW chapter in the continuous growth of the chiropractic narrative established by D.D. Palmer, and developed by his son B.J. Palmer. This will hopefully advance us toward a greater understanding of chiropractic philosophy, chiropractic science, and chiropractic art.

It will develop an explanation of chiropractic that is **hard to vary** giving it a solid foundational platform, that is based on universal principles, of **what is possible ALL OF THE TIME**. It is an invitation for you, the student, to focus on this explanation until the BIG IDEA engages you to make a connection with a larger vision. Sit with it, and if need be, read it again and again and again, until you feel its impact, until you can "see" its larger implications for the world, for history and for you. In other words, until this explanation is transformed from a belief to a knowledge within you. In due time, it will transcend your knowledge and become wisdom. B.J. Palmer wrote,

> *"... Do not fight against receiving the very things you need most. When a new subject is presented for your consideration, study the thing presented, resolve it into knowledge, put it thru a process of analysis and allow time to put it thru a process, which will ripen the knowledge into wisdom, and you will gain many ideas of value. Don't pay so much attention to mere education, to what "the book" says. Be your own judge, put it to the inner test. Concentrate upon knowledge, and you will be overjoyed to find that when the time comes for you to leave the P. S. C. you will be wiser than when you came"*

The Value Of Chiropractic[8: p.19-20]

This concludes the "Note to the student."

FROM PHILOSOPHICAL CONSTRUCTS TO SCIENTIFIC PRINCIPLES

Chiropractic is at a definite turning point in the 2020s. It is moving away from a system of philosophical belief, towards a system of scientific knowledge. It is similar to the distinction between the belief that the earth is flat and the scientific knowledge that the earth is round. (It should be noted that it took several hundred years to shift that paradigm). The reclassification of the 33 principles of chiropractic, from philosophical constructs to scientific axioms, came as something of a complete surprise, and for many, a staggering shock.[7: p.47-51] The response to this surprise re-orientation, from virtually all colors of the chiropractic spectrum, tends to be extreme befuddlement and it is intense. It is because the core issue, which was the limitation of our collective educated intelligence within the context of the past, seems to have breezed over everyone's head except, perhaps, Stephenson himself who recognized that the future would bring further clarification[1: p.55] In other words, our educated intelligence had not yet grown to "see" and understand "WHAT" we now "see" and understand... until today.

In missing this central issue, the leading margin of chiropractic has missed the crucial types of action that are necessary to grow from chiropractic's universal truths. We simply did not "see" these truths as universal scientific truths. Therefore, we used them as our individual personal philosophical truths. It made sense to us; our personal truth became as good as anyone else. I call this phenomenon, the no-truth factor. In other words, your truth is as good as my mine.

One thing has been clear: a profession in which its divisions flat out discredit each other is not a profession that can move forward with any sort of grace, dignity, and integrity. That is exactly where the chiropractic profession finds itself right now. How can we even begin to imagine the future of chiropractic without first recognizing how it has managed to sustain itself for better or for worse for 125 years?

This book is truly a chiropractic re-contextualization that is also a process of rediscovery. The organizing principle is well documented in Stephenson's text but is very little known as the universal truth that it is (see articles 7, 230, 336, 340, 396). This is an eye-opening possibility to witness the power of the chiropractic objective, based on scientific principles that could, in time, literally change the entire world.

INTRODUCTION TO "WHAT"
CHIROPRACTIC IS

My Blue Book, *A New Look at Chiropractic's Basic Science,* reclassifies the 33 principles from philosophical constructs to scientific principles. Among some of the NEW theories that are presented, it demonstrates that force, the second factor of the triune (pri. 4), is information/F. Its function is to unite, through interface, the universal principle of organization and E/matter. Information/F unites the universal principle of organization and E/matter (pri.10).[7: p.53-57] Principle #1 is about the universal principle of organization as Stephenson wrote, "Therefore we are able to go back to the most fundamental principle of all." [1: p.237] This fundamental and universal principle is the starting point of chiropractic. It is an "a priori" statement that cascades into 32 minor principles having for conclusion the chiropractic objective, which is the end point of chiropractic. It is the universal principle of organization that organizes information/F into instructions for the configuration of sub-atomic particles and their velocities **maintaining** them in existence. Instructive information/F is governed by the organizing principle alone. This clarification solves a problem at the foundation of intelligence, namely that the universal principle of organization does NOT create information/F since the laws of conservation of energy, of matter and of information make it impossible. E/matter and information/F are never created and never destroyed. In 2011, it was stated that in the quantum view of the universe, information is never created nor destroyed. It is also verified by principle #5 as it states, in Stephenson's textbook, "In order to have 100% life (universal life) there must be 100% intelligence, 100% force and 100% matter."[1:xxxi] We can state with certainty that the universe is 100%/perfect and complete! The universal principle of organization is a **hard to vary** explanation of how the universe is being **maintained** in existence. This will be further developed later in the text.

Chiropractic principles ALWAYS deal with **what is possible** according to universal laws (pri. 24). To be congruent with this fact, principle #8 is about the function of the universal principle of organization, which is to **organize** information/F into instructions, since the universal laws of conservation prohibit everything from having the function of creating anything at all. Energy, matter and information are never created and never destroyed. Stephenson wrote, "Creation in the brain cell refers to the assembling of something already created, rather than the making of something out of nothing."[1: p.24] Only from a theological standpoint can creation be assumed and theology is NOT chiropractic; theology is beyond the realm of chiropractic. Since, Stephenson clarified that when he used the term creation, it "refers to the assembling of something already created", the term **ORGANIZE** eliminates any conflict that could arise in study. Principle #8 is about the function of an organizing principle. The function of this fundamental and universal principle is to **ORGANIZE** (assemble) information/F into instructions uniting itself to E/matter through organization (pri. 10), thus providing properties and actions to all E/matter to **maintain** it in existence (pri.1). The organized (assembled) information/F is the interface between the organizing principle and E/matter that unites the two (pri.10). It is the instructive input **maintaining** E/matter in existence as an output.

The function of information/F is to unite the universal principle of organization and E/matter (pri.10). Information/F is manifested by motion in E/matter due to the configuration and velocities of its subatomic particles, by the universal principle of organization, thus **maintaining** it in existence (pri.1, 14). It is like the pilot of an aircraft that stays on course throughout the numerous phases of the flight. They are always configuring the aircraft and maintaining the required airspeed, attitude, altitude and situational awareness, all depending upon whether it is the take off phase, the climb phase, the level flight phase, the approach phase, the landing phase, or the touchdown phase. Today, it is possible for any pilot to fly an aircraft and land at its destination if it is equipped with a global positioning system roll steering (GPSS) that interfaces with the composite roll steering commands output by GPS navigators flying a complete, pre-programmed flight plan "hands off" including approach and landing in zero-zero visibility.

In some respects, information/F has a different sort of quality from the two other entities of the triune in terms of describing existence. It is not, for instance, an observable interface. It is what links the other two. Rational logic and sound deductive reasoning, which according to Stephenson is deductive science,[1: p.xvi] is the only means we have to verify that E/matter is **maintained** in existence. We find this similarity in the laws of physics, as conservation laws do for electromagnetic. It underscores, for chiropractors, the congruence of the universal principle of organization in all fields of study. Also, information/F can be moved from one type of medium to another while retaining all its properties. For example, the function of the innate law of living things (innate intelligence) is to compute, codify, characterize, and adapt this information/F for mutual benefit of all the parts of the body. We call that adaptation. The innate law adapts universal information/F and E/matter (pri. 23). It is what makes human capabilities such as coordination of activities of all parts of the body, metabolism, language, and education possible, as well as the possibility of biological adaptability that uses symbolic codes, such as genetic codes and innate impulses.

In addition, the universal principle of organization organizes universal information/F, as the necessary input, to unite E/matter to the organizing principle. The result is an output of motion of E/matter, which **maintains** it in existence (pri. 13, 14, 15). This stands for an attribute with which a physical system, like the universe, is **maintained** in existence. Of course, if universal information/F was adapted by the innate law of living things (ILLT), E/matter would then be alive and would comprise the body of a living thing (pri. 20, 21, 23).

Therefore, the universal principle of organization governs and organizes information/F in order to **maintain** E/matter in existence through motion (pri. 1, 14, 15). The conservation law explains some aspects of motion caused by the universal principle of organization. An important distinction must be made regarding a principle and universal laws. A principle, as defined, is a universal truth that is the foundation of universal laws. As opposed to a universal law, which is based on universal principles. It is defined in teh chiropactic lexicon.

Let us analyze the information used in communication, where the objective is for a receptor to receive a message from a computer through a transmitting medium. For example, the receptor (heart), computer CPU (brain) and transmitter (spinal cord and spinal nerves) are biophysical systems, but the message is not. It is information, initially organized and encoded in the computer CPU, then assembled and propelled in the transmitter, then organized and decoded in the receptor. What is truly amazing, is that, the receptor is able to distinguish the message with perfect reliability from all other messages as long as the receptor is sound, without defects, and that there is no interference within the transmitter, which in the case of the living body is the transmitting neurons, namely the spinal cord and spinal nerves. This perfect reliability gives rise to the principle of coordination (pri. 32) for coherent action of all the parts of the body.

In my book, *A New Look At Chiropractic's Basic Science*, one of the first rather unexpected yields of the reclassification of the 33 principles of chiropractic's basic science has been a new foundational platform on which to reconstruct and reform chiropractic based on the conclusion that chiropractic's basic science clearly reveals the chiropractic objective.[7: p.47-51] We can then scientifically apply the chiropractic objective, based on the 33 principles of chiropractic's basic science.

One of the notorious problems with refining chiropractic, namely that force was considered to be some type of energy that could be measured; that the original triune of life developed by B.J. Palmer regarded force as being measurable through the electroencephaloneuromentiprograph. Many chiropractors to this day don't realize that force, in chiropractic, is non-discrete information (cannot be divided into parts), as opposed to energy, which is discrete due Einstein's equation.[8: p.53-54] When information/F unites E/matter and the universal principle of organization, as one, it becomes the interface, whereas information/F becomes, BOTH, non-discrete and discrete as it instructs the configuration of the electrons, protons, neutrons, and their velocities thus **maintaining** E/matter in existence (pri.1).

Chiropractic has always postulated that in order to do the work that information/F does within the body of living things, such as instructing living E/matter, information/F has to first be non-discrete and non-adapted in order to first **maintain** E/matter in existence. It is through the union of the organizing principle and E/matter, that information/F becomes both non-discrete and discrete. Then the innate law of living things computes, encodes, and adapts the non-material information/F and the material E/matter together; it organizes and assembles universal information/F as innate impulses, which are BOTH, non-discrete and discrete. Information/F unites E/matter with the organizing principle (pri.10). However, information/F is independent of E/matter and the organizing principle. The three aspects of the triune retain their respective identities.

For example: I am writing this book now. Since I exist, it starts as universal information/F, computed, encoded, assembled, and adapted into innate information/F by the innate law due to the fact that I am alive; the innate law is 100% perfect and normal software using the operating system that is the innate brain (field). It is then organized and assembled into innate impulses. My physical brain cells (CPU) are also being adapted to conduct these innate impulses, as code-signals using my nerve cells (transmitters), throughout my body to provide coordination of actions of all my parts (receptors) and presumably complete this book. The body is comprised of organized physical and non-physical systems that continually apply the principles of chiropractic's basic science.

What is this "thing" that has been computed, organized, and adapted in radically different systems of my body and gives rise to their coordinative activities (pri. 32) in writing this book? This is really about instructions from an organizing principle that is now known and proven, in the 2020s. It satisfies the principle of coordination (pri. 32) that is the coherence of biological systems. I mention this because to describe this process you have to refer to the "thing" that has remained unchanged throughout, namely the process, which is only the coded information/F into a non-discrete message rather than any obviously physical E/matter. Why? It is because the message does NOT change. It is the MOMENTUM of the transmission of the message that is interfered with that changes. This is the ONLY "raison d'être" of chiropractic: TO CORRECT SUBLUXATIONS TO RESTORE THE **TRANSMISSION** OF INNATE IMPULSES (pri. 29, 31).

In the 1890s, D.D. Palmer discovered that it is possible for a concussion, where an external invasive information/F overcomes an internal resistive information/F, could cause a vertebral subluxation to occur (pri. 31). This vertebral subluxation causes an interference with the transmission of innate impulse (pri. 29). This, in turn, causes a lack of ease of the transmitting nerve cells, at the site of impingement, thus changing the momentum-flow of transmission of the innate impulse. This lack of ease of the transmitting nerve cells alters the momentum-flow of the innate impulse; it directly violates the principle of coordination causing IN-COORDINATION of DIS-EASE (pri. 30, 32). As we can see, the lack of ease is at the point of contact of the vertebral subluxation within the transmitting E/matter, which is the nerve cells, what Stephenson's calls "local"[1: p.90]. This lack of ease alters the momentum-flow of the transmission of the innate impulse that is constructive toward structural E/matter (pri. 26). This alteration of the momentum-flow reverts it back to a simple nerve impulse and becomes deconstructive toward structural E/matter. Since it is not adapted any longer due to the increase in the limitation of E/matter (pri. 24) it is no longer an innate impulse (with specific momentum-flow), but a nerve impulse (with non-specific momentum-flow) and is deconstructive toward structural E/matter (pri. 26). Stephenson, himself comments that "the 'scrambled' impulse" is no longer a perfectly assembled force of Innate's, it now is practically a common universal force."[1: p. 83]

It is important to note, that the interference with transmission occurs within the transmitting nerve cells and not within the information/F. The non-discrete nature of information/F cannot be altered since it is non-material. It is the momentum-flow of the innate impulse that can be altered and interferes with the "timing" of the input-message of the encoded information/F. The encoded instructive input data is time sensitive. If there is interference with the momentum-flow of the TRANSMISSION of the information/F, the encoded instructive data becomes corrupted. If data corruption occurs, it is ALWAYS going to be within the TRANSMISSION of any computing system. The lack of ease is within the transmitting nerve cells at the point of contact of the vertebral subluxation, what Stephenson calls "local,"[1: p.90] As we saw in the flight analogy, the configuration and velocity of the aircraft is absolutely paramount during every phase of flight. Similarly, it appears that the velocity of the momentum of the motion of subatomic particles plays a crucial role within the expanding universe. That includes the momentum-flow of the innate-impulse.[1: p.96]

As we have clarified, that force in chiropractic is information/F, we will see later on that the law of continuous supply and computation is congruent as we develop a greater understanding of this interference with transmission of innate impulse that we call the vertebral subluxation.

CHIROPRACTIC IS SEPARATE AND DISTINCT FROM EVERYTHING YET IS INCLUSIVE OF EVERYONE

We need to look at the 33 principles until we can see the world with an Above-Down-Inside-Out viewpoint. In my Blue Book, *A New Look at Chiropractic's Basic Science*, it is demonstrated that the 33 principles really constitute chiropractic's basic science and point to a unique organized living system that is SEPARATE and DISTINCT from everything else and that it belongs to EVERYONE due to its ALL INCLUSIVE character. [7: p.53-57]

It also shows how often chiropractors, have substituted the messenger for the message. As a result, chiropractors have spent a great deal of time idolizing the personalities of the people who taught chiropractic and our own egos, trying to get chiropractors and people to idolize us and make a good living at it. Confronted with this reality, I find myself guilty as charged. Too often this obsession became a self-righteous substitute for actually following the governance of the 33 principles of chiropractic's basic science and applying them in practice. We all need to come to grip with this.

On the balance, the response to my Blue Book, *A New Look at Chiropractic's Basic Science*, has been extreme, visceral and quite shocking. The comments that I received were often positively surprising or rather negatively dismissive at first.

Both sides are caught in too narrow a view. There is a bigger picture operating here, and I would like to outline what that might possibly be. I've never heard this particular view that I am about to describe, being expressed by anybody. Stephenson's intuition provided hints. It represents a more inclusive view, and as such can be quite challenging, illuminating, and liberating.

UNDERSTANDING SELF-CORRECTION

Every now and then, nature itself has to adjust its course in light of NEW information on how its way of being is revealing itself. It does so by making various moves that are in effect, a growth that involves self-correcting realignments (e.g., floods, drought, fire, etc.). For a starting point, according to Merriam-Webster, self-correction is "correcting or compensating for one's own errors or weaknesses." The leaders of chiropractic's development are today, in self-correction mode, and have been since the mid-1970s. Three groups emerged, the "non-therapeutic objective straight" movement, also called objective chiropractors (those who EXCLUSIVELY correct VERTEBRAL SUBLUXATIONS, thus practicing EXCLUSIVELY the chiropractic objective, all the time), alongside the "traditional-straight" (those who correct VERTEBRAL SUBLUXATIONS to get sick people well, some of the time), and "mixers" (those who diagnose and add various forms of therapies to get sick people well, some of the time). These three groups form the most populous value systems in our profession today. The confrontational and quite heated battles between them, is known widely as "the political wars." It is based on personal opinions and interpretations of what each think chiropractic is. It has been going on since the first students added their own personal views onto what they learned of chiropractic.

The leaders of chiropractic's development are the objective chiropractors. They practice the chiropractic objective **EXCLUSIVELY.** The chiropractic objective is the conclusion of the 33 principle of chiropractic's basic science, which is to locate, analyze, and facilitate the correction of vertebral subluxations for a normal transmission of innate impulses. Their primary purpose is just that: To be LEADERS of an evolutionary unfolding, what the American psychologist Abraham Maslow called, "a growing tip." This "growing tip" seeks out the most universal, most simple, most inclusive, and most conscious way that is possible at that particular moment and time of chiropractic development. It points to a NEW, novel, creative and adaptive area for the future to unfold into. What kind of future you may ask? Predicting the future of chiropractic, for chiropractors, it is not about what is now. It's about what is next. How our educated intelligence and understanding grow. How our solutions of today's problems will benefit the NEXT generations of chiropractors. How to promote **universal** values and principles to help chiropractors and the people they serve, live their best and most fulfilling lives. How to insure, that people will have access to the correction of vertebral subluxations 5000 years from now. We must first realize that by reducing these universal values into personal values, as we have been doing all along, they have not and will never accumulate into universal change because they attract and legitimize individualists to begin with. Think about that.

PHILOSOPHY -- SCIENCE -- ART

Let us take a long and deep look at chiropractic science (the "WHAT" of chiropractic), which unites chiropractic philosophy (the "WHY" of chiropractic) with chiropractic art (the "HOW" of chiropractic)[1: p.xiv]

Philosophy, science, and art are three separate and distinct aspects of chiropractic. However, D.D. Palmer, B.J. Palmer, and R.W. Stephenson dealt with these three aspects as one and the same.[1: p.xxvii] Of course, D.D. could not develop the science any further than he had, given the knowledge of his time and his death in 1913. We must remember that in 1900, general relativity, quantum physics, computation, and meta-theories had not yet been discovered nor developed.

It was B.J. who continued to develop the philosophy and art of locating, analyzing, and correcting vertebral subluxations. In 1918, B.J. began to take spinographic X-rays and make use of them, along with palpation and nerve tracing, to construct an analysis of the vertebral subluxation. This was followed, in 1922, by the use of the neurocalometer, invented by Dossa Dickson Evans, for pattern work and H.I.O. It was B.J. who also wrote and developed the philosophy from the time he purchased his father's school and business in the early 1900s until his death in 1961. This is how chiropractic was developed over time, from all of the work that was done by the Palmers; this work is a continuous work and **MUST** continue to be developed further. Our chiropractic **task,** therefore, is to **CARRY ON** the further development of their original work. It is for this reason that this book is written for the future students of chiropractic and those chiropractors who still consider themselves students of chiropractic.

We have an "ever growing philosophy comprised of old and new." Rather than seeing "old and new" with a stance of "either/or," the term "ever-growing" acknowledges the **relationship** between the two. We are often surprised to learn that a clearer vision is actually "new" to us now and will be considered "old" by others later on. There is a synergetic **relationship** that can be developed further between philosophy and science. In his book, Professor Alexander Spirkin, vice-president of USSR Philosophical Society wrote, "Science and philosophy have always learned from each other. Philosophy tirelessly draws from scientific discoveries fresh strength, material for broad generalization, which to the sciences it imparts the worldview and methodological impulses of its universal principles". [10: p.42] He goes on to explain why science can't live without philosophy and briefly sketch some domain of intersection of science and philosophy and how the two can have mutual synergy. This certainly applies to chiropractic. Today, we realize that the most important distinction to be understood is between chiropractic's basic science and chiropractic's applied science. "Chiropractic is a philosophy, science, and art".[1: p.xiii] Those are three separate and distinct aspects of chiropractic.

The counterpart to the above statement, that philosophy needs science, basically that the innate law of living things should be the starting point of chiropractic philosophy, is today even a more pressing topic of study for us chiropractors. Too often chiropractic philosophy has been over emphasized at the detriment of chiropractic science and the art of chiropractic.

The job of basic scientists is to discover universal principles that will help us understand life and the world in which we live. That is precisely why I suggested, in 2017, that the 33 principles actually constitute chiropractic's basic science.[7: p.59] Chiropractic's basic science aims at formulating general principles and laws using the universal language of rational logic. It constitutes a systematic organized body of knowledge. As we apply these principles and laws, through chiropractic's applied science, we generate practical methods of locating, analyzing, and facilitating the correction of vertebral subluxations (pri. 31). These methods introduce, more or less, reproducible specific adjustic thrusts with verifiable and falsifiable pre and post checks. This leads us to be able to predict a restoration in transmission of conducted innate information/F (pri. 29, 30) in satisfying the principle of coordination (pri. 32), **ALL THE TIME!!!** Chiropractic's basic science also aims to develop a universal language that enables us to explain the functions of the human body in terms of universal principles and laws that can be falsified or verified by chiropractic research. Chiropractic's basic science enables us to give a **UNIVERSAL** explanation of "WHAT" chiropractic is, that is **hard to vary.**

Conversely, if we do not have a basic science, we are left solely with personal and philosophical interpretations of the 33 principles which would reduce either to speculation, reflecting our lack of knowledge, or be a matter of subjectivity and personal taste, and therefore IRRELEVANT. We would then only infer general statements about the usefulness of the 33 principles for chiropractic from the study of chiropractic's history and by appending that study with a philosophical argument, hence by doing philosophy. This, of course, is what consists of personal truths that widely vary as opposed to **universal truths** that are **hard to vary**. It simply becomes a matter of personal opinion that constitutes the ammunitions supplying the chiropractic wars. This is where we are after 125 years as a profession. Where do we go from here?

TIMED OUT... CHIROPRACTIC

Since this is a task book of error correction and re-contextualization, this next section is organized, similarly to Stephenson's Textbook, following the principles numbered for reference and convenience. Throughout this book, some of the text has been capitalized to emphasize the importance of the content that is revealed as a NEW way of seeing.

Stephenson gives us a definition of science:

> *From Webster's International Dictionary: Accumulated and accepted knowledge which has been systematized and formulated with reference to the discovery of general truths or the operation of general laws; knowledge classified and made available in work, life, or the search for truth; comprehensive, profound, or philosophical knowledge. **Any branch or department of systematized knowledge considered as a distinct field of investigation or object of study.***[1: p.xiv]

From this definition, he goes on to mention, *"Chiropractic is a deductive science"*[1: p.xiv]. "WHAT" chiropractic is, basically, proceeds from a general principle to a specific conclusion. Stephenson also wrote, *"Chiropractic is a radical science. It is a right about face in method and in reasoning"*.
[1: p.xvi]

Further, he wrote, **"The principles of a science are its governing laws. These may be the fundamental truths upon which it is founded, or the governing rules of conduct or operation"**.[1: p. xxix]

Then Dr. Stephenson proceeds to list the principles as follow:

Art. 24.   A LIST OF THIRTY THREE PRINCIPLES, numbered and named.

No. 1. The Major Premise.

> *A Universal Intelligence is in all matter and continually gives to it all its properties and actions, thus maintaining it in existence.*

No. 2. The Chiropractic Meaning of Life.

> *The expression of this intelligence through matter is the Chiropractic meaning of life.*

No. 3. The Union of Intelligence and Matter.

> *Life is necessarily the union of intelligence and matter.*

No. 4. The Triune of Life.

Life is a triunity having three necessary united factors, namely, Intelligence, Force and Matter.

No. 5. The Perfection of the Triune.

In order to have 100% Life, there must be 100% Intelligence, 100% Force, 100% Matter.

No. 6. The Principle of Time.

There is no process that does not require time.

No. 7. The Amount of Intelligence in Matter.

The amount of intelligence for any given amount of matter is 100%, and is always proportional to its requirements.

No. 8. The Function of Intelligence.

The function of intelligence is to create force.

No. 9. The Amount of Force Created by Intelligence.

The amount of force created by intelligence is always 100%.

No. 10. The Function of Force.

The function of force is to unite intelligence and matter.

No. 11. The Character of Universal Forces.

The forces of Universal Intelligence are manifested by physical laws; are unswerving and unadapted, and have no solicitude for the structures in which they work.

No. 12. Interference with Transmission of Universal Forces.

There can be interference with transmission of universal forces.

No. 13. The Function of Matter.

The function of matter is to express force.

No. 14. Universal Life.

Force is manifested by motion in matter; all matter has motion, therefore there is universal life in all matter.

No. 15. No Motion without the Effort of Force.

Matter can have no motion without the application of force by intelligence.

No. 16. Intelligence in both Organic and Inorganic Matter.

Universal Intelligence gives force to both organic and inorganic matter.

No. 17. Cause and Effect.

Every effect has a cause and every cause has effects.

No. 18. Evidence of Life.

The signs of life are evidence of the intelligence of life.

No. 19. Organic Matter.

The material of the body of a "living thing" is organized matter.

No. 20. Innate Intelligence.

A "living thing" has an inborn intelligence within its body, called Innate Intelligence.

No. 21. The Mission of Innate Intelligence.

The mission of Innate Intelligence is to maintain the material of the body of a "living thing" in active organization.

No. 22. The Amount of Innate Intelligence.

There is 100% of Innate Intelligence in every "living thing," the requisite amount, proportional to its organization.

No. 23. The Function of Innate Intelligence.

The function of Innate Intelligence is to adapt universal forces and matter for use in the body, so that all parts of the body will have co-ordinated action for mutual benefit.

No. 24. The Limits of Adaptation.

Innate Intelligence adapts forces and matter for the body as long as it can do so without breaking a universal law, or Innate Intelligence is limited by the limitations of matter.

No. 25. The Character of Innate Forces.

The forces of Innate Intelligence never injure or destroy the structures in which they work.

No. 26. Comparison of Universal and Innate Forces.

In order to carry on the universal cycle of life, Universal forces are destructive, and Innate forces constructive, as regards structural matter.

No. 27. The Normality of Innate Intelligence.

Innate Intelligence is always normal and its function is always normal.

No. 28. The Conductors of Innate Forces.

The forces of Innate Intelligence operate through or over the nervous system in animal bodies.

No. 29. Interference with Transmission of Innate Forces.

There can be interference with the transmission of Innate forces.

No. 30. The Causes of Dis-ease.

Interference with the transmission of Innate forces causes incoordination of dis-ease.

No. 31. Subluxations.

Interference with transmission in the body is always directly or indirectly due to subluxations in the spinal column.

No. 32. The Principle of Coordination.

Coordination is the principle of harmonious action of all the parts of an organism, in fulfilling their offices and purposes.

No. 33. The Law of Demand and Supply.

The Law of Demand and Supply is existent in the body in its ideal state; wherein the "clearing house," is the brain, Innate the virtuous "banker," brain cells "clerks," and nerve cells "messengers."

THE SCIENCE OF CHIROPRACTIC (RECONTEXTUALIZING THE 33)

If you were to ask a basic scientist, "What is your job?" they might answer, "My job is to discover universal principles that help us to better understand life and the world in which we live." Therefore, basic science is about discovering universal principles. Let us see and study those universal principles that we have discovered in chiropractic.

1

No. 1. The Major Premise. A Universal Intelligence is in all matter and continually gives to it all its properties and actions, thus maintaining it in existence.

First of all, we must acknowledge that universal principles belong to the universe and do NOT belong specifically to any particular field of study, including chiropractic. The fact that chiropractors enunciated some principles does NOT give exclusive rights to chiropractic to claim them as its own. For example, the universal law of gravitation is used by physicists, engineers, chemists, pilots, archers, baseball pitchers, etc, etc... Therefore, principle #1 is a universal principle and as such it belongs to anyone wishing to utilize it to find solutions to some of life's problems. However, we must credit D.D. Palmer for being the first person to observe and appropriate this universal principle of organization as a fundamental of chiropractic's basic science, the same way that we credit Isaac Newton for being the first person to observe and appropriate this universal principle of gravity as a fundamental of physics.

D.D. wrote, "Chiropractic is the name of a classified, indexed knowledge of successive sense impressions of biology—the science of life—**which science I created out of principles which have existed as long as the vertebrate**" (emphasis mine).[11: p.1] We must also realize that, in the same way that it is the earth that revolves around the sun and not vice versa, it is the material universe that is within universal principles. The universe is made of material and non-material. The universe is an entity made of physical and nonphysical, discrete and non-discrete. Since there is a whole lot more empty space/time than there is E/matter, it is E/matter that is within space/time. The material is within the non-material. Even Dr. Stephenson in the 1920s had this brilliant insight when he wrote, "Here again we see **embodied IN a principle,** Local and Condition; Local, referring to the **conducting material,** and Condition referring to the functioning -- or **receiving material** (emphasis mine).[1: p.269] We might as well say that it is the **relationship** between the material and the non-material that keeps the universe in existence (pri. 1, 2, 3, 4, 10). This clarification will be extremely useful for a greater understanding of the scientific nature of the principles of chiropractic's basic science.

In my book, *A New Look At Chiropractic's Basic Science*, I mention that as we observe the universe we notice that organization of E/matter has many different and complex levels. Those different and complex levels are governed by a scientific and universal organizing principle.[7: p.17-44] We observe a differentiation of E/matter between living and non-living. A universal and fundamental organizing principle governs all of the different levels of complexity of E/matter in order to continually **maintain** all E/matter in existence all the time. Some of the time through its essential extension, the innate law of living things, it maintains living E/matter alive for a while within the limitations of E/matter (pri. 24). It is for this reason that the chiropractic science constructed by D.D. Palmer, relating to the above quote, continues to be "WHAT" chiropractic truly IS. It is up to the chiropractic profession to promote the truth of "WHAT" chiropractic is, since it belongs to all the people.

The genius of D.D. Palmer, B.J. Palmer, and R.W. Stephenson foresaw that, with time, chiropractic would continually develop, into a forever widening body of knowledge based on NEW facts. This book is a re-contextualization of the 33 principles of chiropractic's basic science. It is based on NEW knowledge that is available in the 2020s that was not available in the 1920s. It is foreseeable that in the future, this re-contextualization will continue to be updated to refine and reflect its truths. Without a doubt, new chapters will be added to the narrative, as chiropractic CONTINUALLY develops into its humanitarian evolutionary approach to life.

In the 1920s, Stephenson wrote, "The Science of Chiropractic holds that a Universal Intelligence created and is maintaining everything in the universe".[1: p.1] This quote is found at the very beginning of the "Freshman Text." He also emphasizes it in the "Senior Text".[1: p. 236]It must be noted that Stephenson's textbook was published fourteen years after the death of D.D. Palmer, the discoverer and founder of chiropractic. It is very well known and documented that D.D. Palmer was using theism as he described universal intelligence. For D.D. Palmer, universal intelligence was the creator of the universe, meaning God. He wrote in his book, "Chiropractic literature makes use of such technical terms as are calculated to enlighten mankind in regard to the Universal Intelligence which the Christian world has seen fit to acknowledge as God. It enables its disciples to recognize the above facts, and teaches them how to adjust their lives accordingly."[11: p.3]

Stephenson appears to continue what D.D. Palmer's original thoughts were about universal intelligence by stating, "in the beginning it created everything." However, intelligence does NOT create the material of the universe. This is prohibited by principle #8, as stated in Stephenson's textbook, "The function of intelligence is to create force." It does NOT create matter, it does NOT create everything; it creates ONLY force. The conservation laws of energy, of matter, and of information make it impossible for anything to be created or destroyed as we studied before. Therefore, it is impossible for a universal intelligence to have "created everything" in the universe. According to Stephenson, "A universal intelligence IS in all matter and continually gives to it all its properties and actions, thus **MAINTAINING** it in existence" (pri. 1).[1: p. xxxi] Principle #1 does NOT state that a universal intelligence creates matter. Principle #1 states that a universal intelligence **IS** (already) included within all E/matter and through its function is to **MAINTAIN** all E/matter in existence!

This is extremely important to clarify and understand. Throughout his textbook, which is approved by B.J. in his letter to "Stevie",[1: p.vii] Stephenson will mention several times that universal intelligence and innate intelligence are scientific principles of organization and coordination (see articles 7, 230, 336, 340, 396). To validate the universal principle of organization he also mentioned, "…but it is not precious as a structure to Universal Intelligence, except insofar as it is a part of the Universal scheme to have structures built in order to tear them down".[1: p. 257] Why this vacillation between theism and scientific principles? Only Dr. Stephenson could answer this question. D.D. Palmer himself asserted with great insight, "That which we may accept as evidence today may not appeal to us as such tomorrow."[11: p.2]

This is where we find ourselves within the second century of chiropractic. As more discoveries and knowledge are shared, we have the moral duty to **CARRY ON** the task of further developing chiropractic as a philosophy, science, and art. This is what we were instructed to do by the discoverer of chiropractic, D.D. Palmer.

With the new knowledge available to us in the 2020s, we realize that E/matter is continually deconstructed and reconstructed due to the re-organization of information/F by the organizing principle. Stephenson wants us look at intelligence whether, universal or innate, as a "mathematical law of nature"[1: p.258] "scientifically, it is the law of organization".[1: p.180] Therefore, let us prove this universal principle of organization scientifically in the laboratory.

For example, let us use the substance known as water (H_2O) that is comprised of two PHYSICAL atoms of hydrogen (H) and one PHYSICAL atom of oxygen (O). The specific momentum of velocities of motion of its subatomic particles (actions) gives rise to the specific configurations of those atoms (properties) forming the molecules of water with the properties and actions of being fluid. It is liquid. Let us pour the liquid water into a copper (Cu) pot over a fire and increase its temperature. We observe that the momentum of velocities and configurations of the molecules of H_2O are changing, thus reorganizing them with the NEW properties and actions of being volatile. It is now vapor. These molecules are still the same two PHYSICAL atoms of hydrogen and one PHYSICAL atom of oxygen but with different properties and actions; this due to their NEW re-organization computed and supplied by the universal principle of organization. The universal principle of organization has re-assembled the information/F into a NEW reconfiguration and a NEW momentum-flow of the velocities of the subatomic particles of the molecules of water in a different way. Now, let us reverse the experiment and instead of having the pot over a fire, let us reduce the temperature of the laboratory down to 0°F, thus reducing the temperature of the water in the pot. Then we observe that the momentum-flow of the velocities and configurations of the molecules of H_2O are changing, thus reorganizing them with the NEW properties and actions of being solid. It is now ice. These molecules are still comprised of the same two PHYSICAL atoms of hydrogen and one PHYSICAL atom of oxygen but with different properties and actions. This is also due to their NEW re-organization computed and supplied by the universal principle of organization that has re-assembled the information/F into a NEW reconfiguration and a NEW momentum-flow of the velocities of the subatomic particles of the molecules of water. We observe through this experiment that E/matter (energy and matter) is never created nor destroyed but always **maintained** in existence by the universal principle of organization (pri. 1). What the universal principle of organization does is compute information/F and organize it with a NEW reconfiguration and a NEW momentum-flow of the velocities of the subatomic particles of E/matter. It is done through the continual re-organization of information/F by the organizing principle that supplies properties and actions to all E/matter (pri. 1, 8). The mathematical equation is:

R_1 (physical reactant) + R_2 (physical reactant) (+/-) ΔE (add or withdraw velocity of physical subatomic particles causing heat/energy) => P (physical product)

$R_1 + R_2 \Delta E = P$

The E/mass of R_1 plus the E/mass of R_2 equals the E/mass of P. With regards to living E/matter, photosynthesis is the prime example of this "mathematical law of nature" since it describes information/F in the form of "electron transfer in a framework based on surface hopping".[12: p. abstract]

This mathematical formula demonstrates that R_1 and R_2 are re-organized into P thus **maintained** in existence congruent with the laws of conservation. It is the sum of the E/mass of reactant 1 plus the E/mass of reactant 2 with an **exchange** of velocity in energy (electrons, protons, and neutrons) that is transformed by the organizing principle; it is thus **maintained** in existence, with different properties, without any E/matter being destroyed or created. There is simply a TRANSFORMATION of E/matter from one state to another due to a change in the velocity of subatomic particles. Nothing is created and nothing is destroyed. The universe ALWAYS remains complete (pri. 5). This mathematical equation is absolute, duplicable, and constant. From this place, we employ deductive reasoning to elaborate on further subsequent principles that **are possible** according to universal laws (pri. 24).

As we empirically verify principle #1, it is crystal clear that principle #1 reveals the governing scientific universal principle of organization. Principle #1 is the initial fundamental principle of chiropractic's basic science. It is the starting point of chiropractic's basic science, its initial condition!

"WHAT" is the nature of this organizing principle of the universe? The answer is found within the interface where the physical and non-physical are united together. It is when E/matter is at any one spot within space and time. It is symbolically, the way that E/matter + organizing principle = existence. The material and non-material are mutually **inclusive** of each other. The link between the two is the "=" sign which is the information/F of the organizing principle **maintaining** the existence of E/matter. Principle #1 evokes the fact that without the organizing principle, E/matter could NOT be **maintained** in existence. The counterpart that the organizing principle could NOT exist without the existence of E/matter is also a fact. ALL of E/matter moves forward through space-time as it is continually **maintained** in existence by the organizing principle. E/matter + organizing principle = existence becomes an equation where there is organized E/matter realm on one side, existence on the other, and the bridge of the "=" sign linking them. Motion is no longer something that happens in space-time, rather motion is simply what we notice when we happen to observe a certain structural form of E/matter within space-time (pri. 14, 15). Our noticing, through observation, reveals that there is the observer and the observed and that they are mutually inclusive of each other. It is "WHAT" makes existence possible. Stephenson wrote, "Our recognition of the intelligence of life or of motion in matter depends upon our ability to recognize law".[1: p.238] Ultimately, it is about observation, awareness and recognition. It is quite shocking to grasp this principle. It seems incredible and almost unthinkable that existence would be dependent on a uniting factor within the triune (pri. 3) and that we would have discovered this link. It really becomes clear that it would have to materialize this way if the equation, E/matter + organizing principle = existence was to be true. The laboratory experiment of water and the observation of photosynthesis attest to its truth. Our observation might be the most important discovery about existence since D.D. Palmer's day. This will be determined by future generations.

What Dr. Stephenson calls the scientific law of organization definitely has a lawmaker as a cause. However, the lawmaker does NOT belong within chiropractic's basic science, the same way that the lawmaker does NOT belong within aviation's scientific principles. It is through chiropractic philosophy, since organization bespeaks intelligence, that we ascribe this cause of the universal principle of organization to a universal intelligence. Chiropractic's basic SCIENCE begins with principle #1 as its starting point, which is comprised of the fundamental scientific universal principle of organization as its description. Principle #1 is the fundamental principle of chiropractic's basic science. It is a statement of the properties and actions of the various states of E/matter, through universal organization, that **maintains** it in existence, and "which will include any and all circumstances that may arise in study".[1: p.xxx]

"Chiropractic is a science of the cause - not effects".[1: p.93] The universal principle of organization CONTINUALLY CAUSES the organization of information/F that supplies properties and actions of all E/matter, thereby **maintaining** it in existence. It is a scientific verified fact! This is principle #1 and it is the starting point of chiropractic's basic SCIENCE.

The properties and actions supplied to E/matter, by the universal principle of organization, are instructive information/F for the configuration and the quantitative velocities of its subatomic particles comprised of electrons, protons, and neutrons that give rise to its structural forms. This universal principle is the beginning of the chiropractic narrative, divided in chapters, including terms such as, universal principle of organization, innate law of living things, triune of existence, limitation of E/matter, information/F, vertebral subluxation, universal cycle, principle of coordination, etc... These terms form descriptions of principles. They are components of the chiropractic narrative. It is the same for the unified field of quantum physics with terms comprising the components of the physics narrative. Some of its terms are proton comprised of "two up quarks and one down quark," neutron comprised of "one up quark and two down quark," "electron, photon, neutrino, quantum wave function, relativity, energy conservation, etc...." So it is for the astronomy narrative with, "planets, galaxies, stars, black holes, quasars, etc...." In the thermodynamics narrative, there are "entropy, first law, second law, etc...." In the biology narrative, there are "DNA, enzymes, phylogeny, ontogeny, etc...." In the electrical engineering narrative, there are "oscillator feedback, vacuum tube amplification, AM-FM radio, and transistors, etc...." And in the computer narrative, there are "software, hardware, programs, applications, processors, data, encoders, decoders, transmitters, etc..." The principles of a field of study are basically sets of divisions about the structure and behavior of field elements. They are names of chapters in the books about the field. Chiropractic is no exception.

Re-contextualized, principle #1 states:

No. 1. THE MAJOR PREMISE.

A UNIVERSAL PRINCIPLE OF ORGANIZATION IS CONTINUALLY SUPPLYING PROPERTIES AND ACTIONS TO ALL E/MATTER, THUS MAINTAINING IT IN EXISTENCE.

2

No. 2. The Chiropractic Meaning of Life. The expression of this intelligence through matter is the Chiropractic meaning of life.

In the 1920s, Stephenson used the word life in principle #2 as *universal life,* to mean existence. He wrote, "The meaning of the term **life** has many interpretations. It is usually accepted to mean existence".[1: p.237] It is actually true since according to principle #1, the universal principle of organization **maintains** E/matter in **existence.** Therefore, chiropractic acknowledges and appropriates principle #1 as the starting point of its basic science. In fact, through rational logic, chiropractic asserts that the expression of this universal principle of organization through E/matter is the chiropractic meaning of existence.

Today, with the new knowledge of the 2020s, we observe principle #1 **maintaining** ALL of E/matter in existence using the equation $(R_1 + R_2 \Delta E = P)$ and we use deductive reasoning. We assert that the supplying of properties of E/matter is the organized information/F by the organizing principle that configures its electrons, protons, and neutrons. We also assert that the supplying of the actions of E/matter is the organized information/F by the organizing principle that imparts the velocities of its electrons, protons, and neutrons. The configurations and velocities of the subatomic particles of E/matter are supplied by the organized information/F into instructions from the universal principle of organization (pri. 1). The organized information/F into instructions by the universal principle of organization (pri. 1) is then expressed by E/matter (pri. 13), and manifested as motion (pri. 14); all governed by the universal principle of organization.

Re-contextualized, principle #2 states:

No. 2. THE CHIROPRACTIC MEANING OF EXISTENCE.

THE EXPRESSION OF THIS ORGANIZING PRINCIPLE THROUGH MATTER IS THE CHIROPRACTIC MEANING OF EXISTENCE.

3

No. 3. The Union of Intelligence and Matter. Life is necessarily the union of intelligence and matter.

In the 1920s Stephenson wrote, "Without intelligence matter could not even exist. Without matter, intelligence could not be expressed".[1: p.238] The function of E/matter is to express information/F (pri. 13). The function of information/F that is organized and governed by the organizing principle (pri. 8) is to unite E/matter to the universal principle of organization (pri. 10) in order to **maintain** E/matter in existence (pri. 1). Stephenson wrote, "our recognition of the intelligence of life or of **motion in matter** (emphasis mine) depends upon our ability to recognize law."[1: p.238]

Today, with the new knowledge of the 2020s concerning the universal principle of organization, we understand that for E/matter to be **maintained** in existence it must continuously be supplied properties and actions through the configuration and velocities of its subatomic particles. It is represented by the equation (F = ma) found in physics. Based on this equation, the action of E/matter is equal to its mass multiplied by the acceleration of its center of mass. E/matter then manifests motion as a result of its existence. It is all about E/matter expressing instructive information/F governed by the universal principle of organization supplying it its properties and actions. These properties and actions are the result of the configuration of electrons, protons, and neutrons with their respective velocities of motion. It is never about expressing the CAUSE but the instructive information of the CAUSE. For example, your father instructs you to help your mother clean the dishes. As you help her clean the dishes, you are NOT expressing your father as CAUSE, but the instructions of your father. It is his instructions that cause you to act. This is an important clarification to make. An entity CANNOT express another entity. An entity can ONLY express the instructive information/F of another entity, for better or for worse. For E/matter to have motion, it must receive instructive information/F from the universal principle of organization. It is this continuous supply of information/F manifested as motion by E/matter (F = ma) that **maintains** it in existence. The **maintaining** of E/matter in existence is actually the union of the organizing principle with E/matter through the interface of information/F.

Re-contextualized, principle # 3 states:

No. 3. THE UNION OF THE PRINCIPLE OF ORGANIZATION AND E/MATTER.

EXISTENCE IS NECESSARILY THE UNION OF THE UNIVERSAL PRINCIPLE OF ORGANIZATION AND E/MATTER.

4

No. 4. The Triune of Life. Life is a triunity having three necessary united factors, namely, Intelligence, Force and Matter.

In the 1920s, Stephenson explains that the bond uniting intelligence and matter is force and cannot be dispensed with.[1: p.238] In those days, Stephenson thought that force was energy as he wrote that, "we perceive force as forms of energy".[1: p.237] He also wrote, **"NOTE: --The term *force* is used in Chiropractic as *energy* is in physics"**[1: p. 253] Joseph B. Strauss wrote, "If we can change matter into pure energy we need to realize that that energy is not the force referred to in our triunity"[13: p.403]

As Einstein's work changed what Faraday and Lavoisier saw, his famous equation of E=mc² makes it crystal clear that energy and matter are interchangeable.[9: p.53-54] It was only in 2017, that the nature of force in chiropractic was identified as information. It is purely non-material. It is non-discrete. It cannot be divided into parts.[7: p.20-21]

Intelligence, force and *matter* are three terms that have been used in Stephenson's textbook to describe the factors comprising the triune of (universal) life, which is truly the triune of existence. He wrote, "the meaning of the term **life** has many interpretations. It is usually accepted to mean existence."[1: p.237] Therefore, the fourth principle is truly about existence. It concerns more specifically the organization of information/F into instructions to supply properties and actions to all E/matter so that it may be **maintained** in existence by the organizing principle. Without the instructive information/F governed by the universal principle of organization, E/matter could not be **maintained** in existence. Conversely, without E/matter, the instructions of the universal principle of organization could not be expressed. Therefore, the instructive information/F expressed by E/matter is the bond ("=") between the organizing principle and E/matter (universal principle of organization + E/matter = existence). The organizing principle, information/F, and E/matter are three factors that are separate and distinct from each other, yet they are united with each other in order for E/matter to be **maintained** in existence. These three factors are separate and distinct from each other. However, it is important to realize that they are deemed EQUALLY necessary for existence to be realize, otherwise we run the risk of emphasizing one over the others. They are separate and distinct entities. Stephenson wrote, "The bond is called force. It is sometimes called 'The Missing Link.' Unlike other sciences, which study them separately, Chiropractic studies them all together."[1: p.238-239] "To study them all together" simply means that they are separate and distinct. It implies that they are EQUALLY necessary for existence to be **maintained**. We will see this more clearly later in this book. There must be differentiation before there can be any possibility of integration. The key is to clearly establish "WHAT" chiropractic is through its SCIENCE; to clearly identify "HOW" to apply its science through its ART; and to clearly explain "WHY" chiropractic does what it does through its PHILOSOPHY. Then we can integrate the three aspects of chiropractic to reconstruct the profession on a solid foundational structure, based on the bedrock of proven scientific principles with an explanation that is **hard to vary.**

Today with the knowledge of the 2020s, when we study chiropractic's basic science we realize that there are two non-discrete (non-material) factors, namely the universal principle of organization and information/F, and one discrete (material) factor, namely E/matter. We have already identified that the term "force," in chiropractic signifies information/F and that it is not physical. This literally means that information/F CANNOT be altered per se, since it is NOT physical. ONLY its TRANSMISSION can be interfered whether it is conducted or it is radiated. The chiropractic objective is **EXCLUSIVELY** to restore TRANSMISSION of **conducted** innate information/F. **"The chiropractor aims only to restore** – to bring about restoration".[1: p.270]

Re-contextualized, principle #4 states:

No. 4. THE TRIUNE OF EXISTENCE.

EXISTENCE IS A TRIUNITY HAVING THREE NECESSARY UNITED FACTORS, NAMELY, THE PRINCIPLE OF ORGANIZATION, INFORMATION/F AND E/MATTER.

5

No. 5. The Perfection of the Triune. In order to have 100% Life, there must be 100% Intelligence, 100% Force, 100% Matter.

In the 1920s, Stephenson understood the limitations in structure of matter. He wrote, " It is obvious that this imperfection is not in matter itself, but in the quantity, quality and arrangement of matter."[1: p. 239] Stephenson also defined "amount" as perfection.[1: p.240] From this moment forward I will use the term "100%/ perfect" to be defined as the perfect amount. It can be found in the lexicon.

Today with the knowledge of 2020's, we realize that $E=mc^2$. Since force, in chiropractic, is information/F, it is the function of information/F that is precisely where the interface occurs. It is the configuration of electrons, protons, and neutrons and their velocities that get to provide the properties and actions of E/matter from the instructions of information/F. This is how E/matter is **maintained** in existence by being continually supplied instructive information/F by the universal principle of organization (pri. 1). In the chiropractic science context, it is the organizing principle that is at work regarding the arrangement of E/ matter through the configuration and velocities of its electrons, protons, and neutrons from **what is possible** according to universal laws within the limits of E/matter (pri. 24). This can be observed through the first law of motion, basically that universal laws are always 100%/perfect by definition, otherwise they would not be universal. It is a proven fact that E/matter is **maintained** in existence by the universal principle of organization. From this empirical observable fact, energy and matter are never created nor destroyed giving rise to the laws of conservation. Those are universal laws; so is limitation of E/matter (pri. 24).

Limitation of E/matter (pri. 24) does not imply imperfection of E/matter, since it is never created nor destroyed. It is within its *structural form* that imperfection occurs. Within ALL formed structures of E/matter is a universal built-in system of deconstruction toward its simple atomic components to be reconstructed as NEW formed structures only to be deconstructed and reconstructed over and over again. This is a universal cycle of existence where the *formed structures* of E/matter are deconstructed and reconstructed again and again FOREVER, so that E/matter is **maintained** in existence (pri. 26). The universe is ALWAYS and FOREVER 100% perfect and complete.

Re-contextualized, principle #5 states:

No. 5. THE PERFECTION OF THE TRIUNE.

IN ORDER TO HAVE EXISTENCE, THERE MUST BE 100%/ PERFECT ORGANIZING PRINCIPLE, 100%/PERFECT INFORMATION/F AND 100%/PERFECT E/MATTER.

6

No. 6. The Principle of Time. There is no process that does not require time.

In the 1920s, Stephenson had enough knowledge concerning time to write, "Since action of matter implies a procession of events, a continuity, naturally time enters into the triunity as an element. Time is an element necessary to the bond between intelligence and matter."[1: p.239] The scientific equation is: $t = d/s$ which means that *time* equals *distance* divided by *speed*.

Today in the 2020s however, the new knowledge of $E=mc^2$ reveals how difficult it is to understand the *concept* of time. Even though we have the equation $t = d/s$, the standard theories of the unified field do not currently address the issue. What we know is that objects behave in ways that show time to be a different kind of dimension pertaining to the motion of E/matter through space. Time is a mathematical continuity where it advances smoothly in flow.[9: p.80-81] This simply means that time is related to space in the universe. It is space/time emerging from the universal principle organizing information/F that configures the subatomic particles of E/matter and their velocities that provide motion to E/matter to **maintain** existence (pri. 1, 6 8, 10, 13, 14, 15).

In the chiropractic science context, we recognize that it is Einstein who was complementing Newton's view of time "flowing uniformly" and called "duration by means of motion".[14: p.23] It must be noted that E/matter exists as a result of its properties and actions being supplied by the universal principle of organization (pri. 1). All E/matter has motion (pri. 14) implying that the configuration of electrons, protons, and neutrons AND their velocities occupy space moving through time (pri. 6). The motion of the particles of E/matter covers distance within space that can be measured and quantified in time ($F = ma$). It is becoming clear why Stephenson mentioned, "Time is an element necessary to the bond between intelligence and matter."[1: p.239] This reveals a new equation in the form of, E/matter = Space/time. The "E" and the "m" of $E=mc^2$ are now just items to go on one side of the "=" sign linking them.[9: p.206] In the equation, E/matter = Space/time, the "=" sign is the organization of information/F.

What is the bond between the organizing principle and E/matter? It is the second factor of the triune, namely, non-discrete information/F.

It is information/F that is the continuous interface or bond uniting the organizing principle to E/matter. Therefore, we observe that within space, time is intrinsic to E/matter in order to be **maintained** in existence by the organizing principle. Remember that principle #1 states: A universal principle of organization *IS CONTINUALLY* supplying properties and actions to all E/matter, thus maintaining it in existence. Time *IS CONTINUALLY* intrinsic to E/matter through the organizing principle; time will ALWAYS be *"an element necessary"* for E/matter to be **maintained** in existence!

Re-contextualized, principle #6 states:

No. 6. THE PRINCIPLE OF TIME.

ALL PROCESSES REQUIRE TIME AND SPACE.

7

No. 7. The Amount of Intelligence in Matter. The amount of intelligence for any given amount of matter is 100%, and is always proportional to its requirements.

In the 1920s, Stephenson's wrote, " 'Amount' means perfection, and that is what is needed for the maintenance of the unit as it is."[1: p.240] All universal principles are absolute and immutable. The way they are formulated may be refined from time to time, however they cannot change otherwise these principles would not be universal in the first place. It is our understanding and use of universal principles that will change and grow. This is because the capability of our educated brain to function is NOT perfect and is continually growing within space/time. This imperfection of the *formed structures* of E/matter is due to its limitation (pri. 24). On the other hand, universal principles are perfect. *Selections from Newton's Principia* states, "a law of motion is a law, not a proposition... It resembles more a statement of something sufficiently clear from experience as not to need a proof."[14: p.31]

Today in the chiropractic science context of 2020, we realize that within the conservation laws, energy and matter is not conserved per se. There is a **RELATIONSHIP** between the two. Within the energy/matter realm, the amount of mass of a particle of E/matter gained in the interaction is ALWAYS going to be BALANCED by an equivalence of energy exchange, what Stephenson calls "Equivalent Vibration." Consequently the sum of mass plus the energy exchanged will ALWAYS remain constant.[1: p.300, 326] It is the reason WHY, within the equation $E=mc^2$, the "E" can become "m" and "m" can become "E." It is ALWAYS 100%/PERFECT and complete. The universal principle of organization is 100%/perfect and it is absolute (pri. 5).

Re-contextualized, principle #7 states:

No. 7. THE PERFECTION OF THE ORGANIZING PRINCIPLE IN E/MATTER.

THE PERFECTION OF THE ORGANIZING PRINCIPLE FOR ANY PARTICLE OF E/MATTER IS ALWAYS 100%/PERFECT AND COMPLETE.

CONSERVATION OF ENERGY, OF MATTER, AND OF INFORMATION

Before we continue with principle #8 of chiropractic's basic science, we must clarify an important fact. As mentioned before, principle #8 makes it impossible for universal intelligence to have created everything in the universe since, according to Stephenson's "the function of intelligence is to create force" (pri. 8). I would add that the function of universal intelligence is **"ONLY"** to create universal information/force. I demonstrated above that force, in chiropractic, is information/F and NOT energy due to $E=mc^2$ which makes energy and matter interchangeable (same particles with different properties and actions). We do know the universal law of conservation of matter and the universal law of conservation of energy, whereas energy and matter are never created nor destroyed. Chiropractic is ALWAYS about **what is possible** according to universal laws (pri. 24).

How about information? Is information subject to the universal laws of conservation? The answer is an emphatic YES! It was experimentally proven in 2007, by the discovery of the "no hiding theorem" documented at PhysOrg.com,[15: p.1] "Now for the first time, a team of physicists consisting of Pati, along with Jharana Rani Samal (deceased) and Anil Kumar of the Indian Institute of Science in Bangalore, India, has experimentally tested and confirmed the no-hiding theorem." The physicists have published their study on the no-hiding theorem test in a recent issue of *Physical Review Letters.*[16] The work is dedicated to the memory of Samal, who died in November 2009 on her 27th birthday and who performed all of the experimental work of the paper.

"In the classical world, information can be copied and deleted at will. In the quantum world, however, **the conservation of quantum information means that information cannot be created nor destroyed**. This concept stems from two fundamental theorems of quantum mechanics: the no-cloning theorem and the no-deleting theorem"[15: p.1]

A third and related theorem, called the no-hiding theorem, addresses information loss in the quantum world. According to the no-hiding theorem, if information is missing from one system (which may happen when the system interacts with the environment), then the information is simply residing somewhere else in the Universe; in other words, the missing information cannot be hidden in the correlations between a system and its environment. Physicists Samuel L. Braunstein at the University of York, UK, and Arun K. Pati of the Harish-Chandra Research Institute, India, first proved the no-hiding theorem in 2007. Until now, however, the no-hiding theorem had been a purely theoretical concept.

This NEW knowledge introduces us to the extremely important NEW fact that information/F is subject to the universal laws of conservation and cannot be created nor destroyed. It is consistent with principle #5 revealing that the universe is 100%/perfect and complete.

8

No. 8. The Function of Intelligence. The function of intelligence is to create force.

In the 1920s, Stephenson's deductive reasoning regarding the function of intelligence was based on his understanding of "force as being some form of energy," as he wrote, **"NOTE: -- The term force is used in Chiropractic as energy is in physics"**.[1: p.253] This is NOT true today. This statement of terms is NOT consistent with $E=mc^2$. However, remember that Stephenson was also equating universal intelligence with God. As you recall, he wrote, "The Science of Chiropractic holds that a Universal Intelligence **created** and is maintaining everything in the universe" (emphasis mine).[1: p.1] We must understand that for Dr. Stephenson it was logical and reasonable for him to say that the function of intelligence was to create everything since for him, "A Universal Intelligence CREATED and is maintaining EVERYTHING in the universe" (emphasis mine). Therefore, since he viewed universal intelligence as being synonymous with God, according to him, the function of universal intelligence/God would be to create everything, and that would obviously include force. We must always remember that D.D. and B.J. and Stephenson were writing with the knowledge they had within the context of the 1920s. We must never lose sight of this truth.

The conservation laws prohibit energy from EVER being created or destroyed by anything, including "a mathematical law of nature"[1: p.258] or a "law of organization",[1: p.180] unless of course one equates "universal intelligence" to be God. We have already established that theology is the study of God with numerous religious beliefs and that theology is beyond the realm of chiropractic. "Chiropractic is a philosophy, science and art."[1: p.xiii] Furthermore, it is principle #24 that points to the fact that intelligence cannot break a universal law due to the limitation of E/matter. This is simply due to the reality that universal laws are immutable, unchangeable and absolute. Universal laws cannot be broken (pri. 5, 7). Chiropractic's basic science is based ONLY on **what is possible** according to universal laws ALL THE TIME (pri. 24) and that includes the laws of conservations. Therefore, principle #8 CANNOT be about creating anything (including force). Only from a theological perspective, that a universal law could be overruled by the LAWMAKER. Chiropractic does not address this issue. It is beyond the realm of chiropractic. Chiropractic is NOT theology. Chiropractic is philosophy, science and art.[1: p.17]

Today in the 2020s, we indentified force in chiropractic to be information/F. We clarified and refined its nature through observation and experimentation.[17] Since information/F can never be created nor destroyed,[16] what is the function of "intelligence"? Could it be found within, what Stephenson himself called, "scientifically, it is the law of organization"?[1: p.180] He said that universal intelligence was, "... but as a mathematical law of nature."[1: p.258] Stephenson is correct in asserting that universal intelligence is a scientific universal principle of organization. As such, this universal principle of organization continually **organizes** information/F that is never created nor destroyed,[16] providing properties and actions to all E/matter, thus **MAINTAINING** it in existence (pri. 1).

In the chiropractic science context, the universal principle of organization (UPO) governs information/F, **organizing** them into instructions that supply properties and actions to all E/matter. It is the universal principle of organization that **organizes** information/F into instruction that, in turn, configures the subatomic particles of E/matter and governs their velocities (F = ma). This function gives rise to infinite possibilities and potentialities of structural forms of E/matter. The configuration and velocities of the subatomic particles are actually manifested by the second universal law of motion,[14: p.29] (pri. 14, 15). It is a direct effect that is CAUSED by the universal principle of organization, thus **maintaining** E/matter in existence (pri. 1). The motion of electrons, protons and neutrons is such that each atom is almost entirely empty space.[9: p.99] This empty space within each atom is non-discrete. The universal principle of organization is non-discrete also and it **organize**s information/F into instructions, supplying properties and actions for E/matter to be **maintained** in existence. It is clear that it is the function of organizing information/F into instructions, by the organizing principle, that unites this organizing principle to E/matter, thereby **maintaining** it in existence (pri. 1, 8). The organizing of information/F is actually the function of the organizing principle.

Re-contextualized, principle #8 states:

No. 8. THE FUNCTION OF THE PRINCIPLE OF ORGANIZATION.

THE FUNCTION OF THE PRINCIPLE OF ORGANIZATION IS TO ORGANIZE INFORMATION/F.

9

No. 9. The Amount of Force Created by Intelligence. The amount of force created by intelligence is always 100%.

In the 1920s, Stephenson defined the term *amount* as perfection[1: p.240] and wrote that, "Force is an immaterial thing."[1: p.250] We also know that the universal principle of organization is non-material meaning that it is non-discrete. It organizes information/F into instruction that supplies properties and action to E/matter, giving rise to unlimited possibilities and potentialities of configurations, and velocities of the subatomic particles of E/matter, thus **maintaining** it in existence. Energy/matter, on the other hand, is material ($E=mc^2$) meaning that E/matter is discrete. From the above statement from Stephenson, we understand that information/F is non-discrete and is organized by the organizing principle that is also non-discrete.

Stephenson defined "amount" as perfection. Rational logic reveals that the non-material cannot be quantified, therefore the use of the expression "100%/perfect" is appropriate for principle #9.

Today, in the 2020s, we assert that non-discrete 100%/perfect information/F is NOT created by universal intelligence or the universal principle of organization; that is prohibited by the law of the conservation of information.[16] It is also prohibited by principle #24, which states "... as long as it can do so WITHOUT (emphasis mine) breaking a universal law." Non-discrete 100%/perfect information/F is organized into 100%/perfect instructions by the non-discrete 100%/perfect principle of organization supplying properties and actions to every subatomic particle in the universe. In 1932, Ernest Rutherford was the first to discover that the atom was almost entirely empty space. Then Enrico Fermi, in 1934, observed that the nucleus of the atom is comprised of the neutron that could go in and out of the atom.[9: p.99] This observation reveals that the motion of electrons, protons, and neutrons of the atoms, supplied by the instructive information/F of the universal principle of organization, is a configuration that gives rise to the properties of the particles of E/matter and that their velocities give rise to the actions of the particles of E/matter. In other words, it is the continuous motion of E/matter manifesting 100%/perfect instructive information/F from the UPO that is **maintaining** E/matter in existence (pri. 1, 14, 15). ONLY a 100%/perfect organizing principle can continually achieve this.

Re-contextualized, principle #9 states:

No. 9. THE AMOUNT OF INFORMATION/F.

THE INFORMATION/F ORGANIZED BY THE PRINCIPLE OF ORGANIZATION IS ALWAYS 100%/PERFECT.

10

No. 10. The Function of Force. The function of force is to unite intelligence and matter.

In the 1920s, Stephenson wrote, "Structures of matter cannot exist without the building forces of intelligence. Structure of matter cannot continue to exist without the **maintenance** by intelligence."[1: p.251] For example, the composition E/matter that we call water is H_2O; it cannot be **maintained** in existence without information/F that is **organized** into instructions by the organizing principle.

In the chiropractic science context, the structures of discrete E/matter are **maintained** in existence by the non-discrete universal principle of organization. The atoms forming the structures of E/matter require continuous configurations and velocities in order for E/matter to be **maintained** in existence. It is the motion of electrons, protons, and neutrons within the atom that **maintains** its existence (pri. 14, 15). Therefore, it is non-discrete information/F **organized** into instructions by the non-discrete universal principle of organization that **unites** E/matter and the organizing principle. This union is the actual interface of the non-discrete with the discrete, the non-material with the material, the non-physical with the physical. The **maintaining** of E/matter in existence requires the union of E/matter with the organizing principle. This union of the organizing principle and E/matter is the function of information/F. The universal principle of organization governs information/F that **unites** E/matter to the organizing principle itself. It is a wider principle dealing with all E/matter being kept in existence as it is united to the universal principle of organization. The **organized** information/F = **maintenance** of E/matter in existence. The "=" sign is the linking of these two realms. It is the union of the material with the non-material. It is the function of non-discrete information/F governed by the non-discrete organizing principle INTERFACING with discrete E/matter and that unites the two. It is the bridge of "=" linking them. What is revealed is astonishing. Every particle of E/matter is **maintained** in existence manifesting motion governed by the organizing principle (pri. 1, 14, 15). Existence is something that happens through the interface. It is simply what we notice when we happen to be observing E/matter with a particular configuration of properties and action. In scientific circles this is called epigenetic. According to Christopher Kent, DC, ACP, JD, "The take home-message is stunning. Epigenetic signals from the environment can be passed on from one generation to the next, sometimes for several generations, without changing a single gene sequence... For the chiropractor, correction of nerve interference takes on a deeper significance."[18] This means that what we think, say, or do (or don't think, don't say or don't do) affects future generations, since we relate to each other, directly or indirectly. This of course is manifested whether we like it or not, want it or not, believe it or not (pri. 17). So, it is your choice, as chiropractors, and it is significant! The aim of locating, analyzing, and facilitating the correction of vertebral subluxation is the restoration of transmission of conducted innate information/F (pri. 29, 30, 31,) satisfying the principle of coordination (pri. 32), which underscores its universal humanitarian approach to life. Philosophically, it is like asking the questions, "When a tree falls in the forest, does it make a noise if there is no one to hear it?" Or, "Without an observer, does E/matter exist?" The observer and the observed are intrinsic to one another. They are one and the same.

Today, with the knowledge available to us in the 2020s, "Energy does not stand alone, and neither does mass. But the sum of mass plus energy will always remain constant".[9: p.54] Energy and mass are one and the same! Stephenson wrote, "The purpose of mental impulses is Innate balance or control of universal forces, which are always in the tissue cell."[1: p.202] E/matter is **maintaine**d in existence by the universal principle of organization that continually supplies its properties and actions by organizing the configurations and velocities of its subatomic particles (pri.1, 8). The universe is always balanced, never created, never destroyed, always maintained in existence!

Re-contextualized, principle #10 states:

NO. 10. THE FUNCTION OF INFORMATION/F.

THE FUNCTION OF INFORMATION/F IS TO UNITE THE PRINCIPLE OF ORGANIZATION AND E/MATTER.

11

No. 11. The Character of Universal Forces. The forces of Universal Intelligence are manifested by physical laws; are unswerving and unadapted, and have no solicitude for the structures in which they work.

In the 1920s, Stephenson wrote in the senior section of his textbook, "[universal forces] are antipodal to adapted forces… It is but the working of the great cycle…"[1: p.251] He also wrote, "Dr. Palmer holds that… 'The law of a universal cycle is absolute'."[1: p.336] It is true that this law of universal cycles consists of a continuous organization of information/F that is supplied as input to be computed by an organizing principle and expressed as output, by E/matter (pri. 13). The law of the universal cycle of existence functions through construction, deconstruction, and reconstruction (order, disorder, reorder) (pri. 26).

Today, with the NEW knowledge of the 2020s, we realize that the universe can be described in terms of CONTINUAL expanding transformation, using the equation "$R_1 + R_2 \, \Delta E = P$". There is an important distinction regarding a principle and universal laws. **A principle is a fundamental truth that serves as the foundation of universal laws.** For example, the universal principle of organization continuously **organizes** information/F into instructions supplying properties and actions to E/matter that are manifested by motion as a physical law ($F = ma$). Thus, transformation requires deconstruction and reconstruction of E/matter for re-organization to be manifested as motion (pri. 14, 15) from the universal principle of organization in order to **maintain** E/matter in existence (pri. 1). This is a fundamental truth. Here is a schematic formula to describe this continuous cycle (The sign "$\rightarrow$" signifies the unification of E/matter to the organizing principle):

Organized instruction input $\rightarrow$ Computing = Motion output of E/matter.

The organizing principle continually **organizes** information/F into continuous input/instructions that are continually computed, and then expressed by E/matter as a continuous output/motion manifested through physical laws (pri. 1, 8, 10, 13, 14, 15). This is precisely from the non-discrete instructive information/F that the non-discrete universal principle of organization is united to discrete E/matter in order to maintain it in existence, as it is re-organized through reconstruction and deconstruction ($R_1 + R_2 \, \Delta E = P$). The interface of existence IS instructive information/F from the organizing principle EXPRESSED by

E/matter (pri. 13) and manifested through motion (pri. 14) as physical laws. For example, two atoms of hydrogen + one atom of oxygen = a molecule of water. The "+" sign is the instructive information/F input **organized** by the universal principle of organization. The "+" sign is the interface maintaining water in existence. The "=" sign is the output expression of instructive information/F by E/matter that is manifested as the properties and actions of water (pri. 8, 10, 13, 14). This equation $(R_1 + R_2 \Delta E = P)$ applies to EVERY particle of E/matter in the universe.

Re-contextualized, principle #11 states:

NO. 11. THE CHARACTER OF UNIVERSAL INFORMATION/F.

THE INFORMATION/F OF THE UNIVERSAL PRINCIPLE OF ORGANIZATION ARE MANIFESTED BY PHYSICAL LAWS; ARE UNSWERVING AND UNADAPTED, AND HAVE NO SOLICITUDE FOR THE STRUCTURES IN WHICH THEY WORK.

12

No. 12. Interference with Transmission of Universal Forces. There can be interference with transmission of universal forces.

In the 1920s, the prevailing conception was that force was some "form of energy".[1: p.253] Energy can be interfered with in many ways. For example, an umbrella shades you from the sun on the beach, or lead apron interferes with X-ray exposure, etc. However, with E=mc², we know that energy and matter are interchangeable and we have since discovered that force in chiropractic is information, thus the term information/F.[7: p.20]

Today, in the 2020s, we have NEW knowledge acquired from computation and quantum fields. The transmission of coded data (information/F) can be interfered with through transmitters. "Interference may prevent reception altogether, may cause only a temporary loss of signal, or may affect the quality of the sound or picture produced by your equipment. The two most common causes of interference are transmitters and electrical equipment".[19] Since instructive information/F can travel in radiated forms it can be interfered with by counter-information/F, for example the previously umbrella interfering with sunrays. Therefore, within the scientific context of today's knowledge, we assert that the transmission of universal information/F from a source through a medium, in the form of conduction or radiation, to a receiver is subject to interference. In other words, the transmissions of instructive information/F from the organizing principle to E/matter can be interfered with.

Re-contextualized, principle #12 states:

No. 12. INTERFERENCE WITH UNIVERSAL INFORMATION /F.

THERE CAN BE INTERFERENCE WITH THE TRANSMISSION OF UNIVERSAL INFORMATION/F.

13

No. 13. The Function of Matter. The function of matter is to express force.

Once again, in the 1920s, the prevailing conception was, according to Stephenson, **"The term force is used in Chiropractic as energy is in physics"**.[1: p.253] Now it is revealed, from $E=mc^2$, that energy and matter are interchangeable, being comprised of the same physical particles of matter with different configurations and velocities. Therefore, force CANNOT be energy otherwise the triune would be the organizing principle (intelligence), energy/matter (force), energy/matter (matter). This assemblage would devolve the triune into a duality whereas force and matter would be the same. This is NOT possible due to principle #4 stating that, "existence is a *triunity* having **THREE** necessary united factors". [1: p.xxxi] This would collapse the central core of chiropractic, namely, that it is possible for interference to alter the transmission of the non-discrete uniting factor (called information/F), where it is possible for its transmission to sustain interference due to vertebral subluxation. Remember that chiropractic is about **what is possible** according to universal laws. Chiropractic is about **what is possible** ALL THE TIME without breaking a universal law (pri. 24).

Information/F is non-discrete (non-physical); its function is to unite. Once again, force, in chiropractic, is non-discrete information/F **organized** by the universal principle of organization uniting it to E/matter (pri. 8, 10). This is the interface of the non-discrete (non-material) realm with the discrete (material) realm. This is precisely where the material and the non-material meet, **maintaining** all the content of the universe in existence giving rise to the conservation laws of Faraday, Lavoisier, and Samal, et al. It is this universal principle of organization that explains the conservation laws of matter, energy and information ($R_1 + R_2 \Delta E = P$); it also **maintains** existence (organizing principle + E/matter = existence. The "=" sign is the link between the organizing principle and E/matter. The universal principle of organization, in chiropractic, is fundamental and becomes the starting point of chiropractic's basic science. It is the bedrock of the foundational platform of everything chiropractic. Through deductive reasoning using rational logic, 32 subsequent principles form the foundational structure of an evolutionary humanitarian service called chiropractic!

Today, in the 2020s, it is accurate to state that the function of discrete E/matter is to express non-discrete information/F. The function of discrete E/matter is a continuous result of being **maintained** in existence through the uniting factor, which is 100%/perfect information/F that is **organized** by a 100%/perfect/universal principle of organization. It is the function of E/matter to physically reveal the uniting function of non-physical information/F by specifically expressing information/F that **maintains** it in existence (pri. 10, 13). At this precise moment, information/F is transformed in both material and non-material, through its being expressed by E/matter (pri. 13). Through the function of E/matter we observe the transformation of non-discrete information/F as it unites (bonds) the organizing principle with E/matter. It is exactly when E/matter expresses information/F that it has morphed into "discrete/non-discrete" (material/non-material); and that is how the universal principle of organization is **maintaining** ALL the physical particles of the universe in existence.

Within the chiropractic science context, E/matter expresses information/F as its function (pri. 13). This information/F is instructive to E/matter supplying its properties and actions continually governed by the function of the organizing principle (pri. 1, 8) through deconstruction and reconstruction. This is the way that existence is continually **maintained.** For example, if you come to a stop sign and you stop your car, you are expressing the instructive information/F of the red and white code (sign) "S-T-O-P". You are NOT expressing the WHOLE law of traffic, only the instructive information/F regarding this particular road to keep the flow of traffic safe at this specific intersection. You are NOT expressing the lawmaker either. You do not even know the lawmaker, the one WHO chose to put a stop sign at that intersection, on that particular road, in that particular country, in that particular state, in that particular city. All you are expressing is the instructive information/F of stopping your car at that particular stop sign. Another example could be if your father asked you to help your mom clean the dishes. You were NOT expressing your father as you cleaned the dishes. You were expressing his request, his intent in the form of instructive information/F.

Re-contextualized, principle #13 states:

No. 13. THE FUNCTION OF E/MATTER.

THE FUNCTION OF E/MATTER IS TO EXPRESS INFORMATION/F.

14

No. 14. Universal Life. Force is manifested by motion in matter; all matter has motion, therefore there is universal life in all matter.

In the 1920s, Stephenson clarified the word life to mean existence. Yet, he used the word universal life rather than existence for principle #14. However, according to Newton's law of motion, every particle of E/matter has motion (F = ma).[14: p.29] This is due to the universal principle of organization continually governing instructive information/F and supplying properties and action to E/matter **maintaining** it in existence (pri. 1). In the universe, we have evidence of this reality as we observe complex organization patterns in various states of E/matter. The organizing principle governs EVERY different level of organization of E/matter, all of them, no exclusion! It is the same 100%/perfect principle at work within atoms, molecules or compounds, cells, organs, systems, and bodies. It simply reflects more complex patterns of organization.

Today, in the 2020s, E=mc^2 reveals that force CANNOT be energy. In chiropractic, we recognize force as being information/F that is expressed by E/matter (pri. 13). EXISTENCE IS NECESSARILY THE UNION OF THE UNIVERSAL PRINCIPLE OF ORGANIZATION AND E/MATTER (pri. 3). Existence is thus revealed through E/matter expressing the information/F governed by the organizing principle. What is the manifestation of the function of E/matter? It is the actual motion (F = ma) of ALL of its physical particles. That is HOW we can actually "see," "observe" "perceive" and "sense" existence! Remember existence is simply what we notice when we happen to be looking at E/matter with a particular configuration of properties and action at a certain spot within space-time.

Within the context of chiropractic science, the electrons, protons, and neutrons continually move while forming infinite configurations and velocities of atoms forming unlimited structures of E/matter. All E/matter has motion therefore all E/matter has existence. Once again, we see that it is the universal principle of organization, in principle #1, that **maintains** all E/matter in existence!

Re-contextualized, principle #14 states:

No. 14. EXISTENCE.

INFORMATION/F IS MANIFESTED BY MOTION IN E/MATTER; ALL E/MATTER HAS MOTION, THEREFORE ALL E/MATTER HAS EXISTENCE.

15

No. 15. No Motion without the Effort of Force. Matter can have no motion without the application of force by intelligence.

In the 1920s, Stephenson's educated intelligence (the capability of his educated brain to function) was a prisoner of his time, the same way that our educated intelligence is a prisoner of our time in the 2020s. We can only understand with the knowledge that is available to us within the timeframe and context of our life. Those that will come after us will have more knowledge and will be able to **carry on** the continuous development of chiropractic in a way that we cannot realize at this moment in time. Stephenson formulated and organized the 33 principles that had been discovered by D.D. Palmer and his son B.J. Palmer with his educated intelligence, according to his specific knowledge, when he published the *Chiropractic Text Book* in 1927. We know that Stephenson thought that force was some kind of energy. He posited that the cause of the motion of E/matter was energy. However, since the establishment of $E=mc^2$, we comprehend that energy and matter are one and the same with different velocities of subatomic particles. Therefore, the cause of motion cannot be energy. It has to be something totally different and distinct from energy/matter.

Today, with the new knowledge of the 2020s, we realize that energy and matter are interchangeable within the parameters of $E=mc^2$. In the context of chiropractic science, we have also identified force, in chiropractic, as information/F that is organized into instructions by the organizing principle. It is specific instructive information/F, governed by the universal principle of organization, that CAUSES E/matter to have continuous motion, to have properties and actions. Newton called this phenomenon "Motive force" ($F = ma$) and "is defined as taking place 'in a given time'." $t = d/s$ [14: p.30] Stephenson also wrote, "An act is an intangible thing and it is never perceptible to us, unless matter makes it so."[1: p.255] We can see that the CAUSE for E/matter to act is instructive information/F **organized** by the universal principle of organization. Action is motion ($F = ma$). This motion is, ultimately, the manifestation of information/F in E/matter (pri. 14) thus **maintaining** it is existence (pri. 1).

Re-contextualized, principle #15 states:

No. 15. NO MOTION WITHOUT INSTRUCTIVE INFORMATION/F.

E/MATTER CAN HAVE NO MOTION WITHOUT INSTRUCTIVE INFORMATION/F SUPPLIED BY THE PRINCIPLE OF ORGANIZATION.

16

No. 16. Intelligence in both Organic and Inorganic Matter. Universal Intelligence gives force to both organic and inorganic matter.

In the 1920s, Stephenson simply stated the obvious. However, as we look closely at the natural world, we observe various states of E/matter and of different levels of complex organization (atoms, molecules, compounds, cells, tissues, organs, systems, bodies, etc...). These different levels of organization are the result of the properties and actions of E/matter supplied from the instructive information/F organized and governed by the universal principle of organization. Organic E/matter is basically the same as inorganic E/matter, except that organic E/matter is ORGANIZED with at least one or more atoms of carbon. Within the more complex levels of organization of living E/matter we observe the unique ability of organic E/matter to be adaptable to stimuli and to respond to it. Universal instructive information/F supplied by the universal principle of organization and organized into more complex levels of organization of living E/matter are now computed, coded, and adapted by the innate law of living things for use in the body (pri. 23).

Within the chiropractic science context, the electrons, protons, and neutrons of E/matter are continually supplied instructive information/F **organized** by the universal principle of organization that is governing their configurations and velocities. These give rise to different levels of complex structural forms to both inorganic and organic E/matter. Organic E/matter is adaptable due to the innate law of living things (pri. 23).

We know that organic E/matter always contains carbon atoms, forming organic compounds that include nucleic acids, found in DNA, lipids and, fatty acids found in the cells. Also found in the cells are proteins and enzymes necessary for cellular processes to be computed and more. Living E/matter is comprised of the same elemental particles as non-living E/matter. It is organized into structures by the instructive information/F of the organizing principle that has been adapted by the innate law of living things, which is an essential extension of the organizing principle governing living E/matter. Meanwhile, non-living E/matter includes inorganic compounds including salt, metals, and other elemental atoms and molecules. ALL compounds (inorganic and organic) undergo deconstruction and reconstruction depending upon the instructive information/F organized and governed by the universal organizing principle and the innate law of living things.

Today in the 2020s, we understand that the movement toward more complex levels of organization of E/matter gives rise to a broad universal field. This field is formed from inorganic levels of divided E/matter, to inorganic levels of condensed E/matter, to organic levels of active organization and living E/matter, onto levels of thinking E/matter, up the ladder of complexity. We are observing the motion ($F = ma$) of all the particles E/matter, both organic and inorganic, due to the instructive information/F from the universal principle of organization (pri. 15). This motion of organic and inorganic E/matter is the manifestation of E/matter being **maintained** in existence (pri. 1).

Re-contextualized, principle #16 states:

No. 16. ORGANIZATION IN BOTH INORGANIC AND ORGANIC E/MATTER.

A PRINCIPLE OF ORGANIZATION GOVERNS BOTH ORGANIC AND INORGANIC E/MATTER.

Being at the half waypoint of the 33 principles of chiropractic's basic science, we are introduced to living E/matter (biological) revealing that at each level of increasing complexity, NEW structures emerge that do not exist at lower levels. These NEW structures of E/matter, at the higher levels of complexity, are comprised of the same electrons, protons, and neutrons as the lower levels. They simply express different instructive information/F that are governed by the same organizing principle in order to be **maintained** in existence. Therefore, the levels of increasing complexity are deducible from but not reducible to the lower levels of complexity. The CAUSE of such a broad trajectory is found within the universal principle of organization.

17

No. 17. Cause and Effect. Every effect has a cause and every cause has effects.

In the 1920s, Stephenson possessed the knowledge necessary to include this universal principle just before introducing the innate principles. He wrote, "The study of Chiropractic is largely a study of the relations between Cause and Effect, and Effect and Cause".[1: p.256]

Understanding the relationship between cause and effect requires us to philosophically examine the CAUSE, the SOURCE of the universal principle of organization. The starting point of chiropractic's basic science is principle #1, namely, A UNIVERSAL PRINCIPLE OF ORGANIZATION IS CONTINUALLY SUPPLYING PROPERTIES AND ACTIONS TO ALL E/MATTER, THUS MAINTAINING IT IN EXISTENCE. The verb "IS" denotes an intrinsic presence of the organizing principle CONTINUALLY supplying properties and actions. It is an ACT as Stephenson calls it.[1: p.255] Furthermore, it is a **CONTINUAL** ACT that **maintains** E/matter in existence. The ACT in principle #1 is the universal principle of organization. It is the CAUSE of the effect of E/matter being **maintained** in existence (pri.1), thus manifesting motion (F = ma) (pri. 14). An ACT logically requires an ACTOR that would be the CAUSE of a cause! The CAUSE of organization is the universal principle of organization. It is the starting point of **chiropractic's basic science** and comprises the "WHAT" of chiropractic! This begs the question, "What is the CAUSE of the universal principle of organization?" To answer this question, we must rely on chiropractic philosophy, which is the "WHY" of chiropractic. Chiropractic consists of three aspects, namely, philosophy, science, and art.

The universal principle of organization is an ACT organizing information/F into instructions that supply properties and actions to E/matter in order to **maintain** it in existence (pri. 1). It is the core assumption and the starting point of chiropractic's basic science where everything else derives its universal values. It is the a priori statement of chiropractic that is assumed to be true from empirical observation. It is a proven fact of laboratory experiments. It is the first principle of **chiropractic's basic science.** It is the central reference point from which 32 subsequent principles of chiropractic's basic science are derived. Using chiropractic philosophy, with rational logic, we assert that organization bespeaks intelligence, that there cannot be organization without intelligence. Intelligence is intrinsic to organization. "The intelligence function comprises the gathering, evaluation and dissemination of information."[20: p. 365] Therefore, universal organization bespeaks universal intelligence. The universal principle of organization is non-discrete and so is the universal intelligence intrinsic to it, also non-discrete. Philosophically, this universal intelligence is the CAUSE of the universal principle of organization that is the CAUSE of the **organization** of the universe. It is this organizing principle that is **maintaining** E/matter in existence (pri. 1). This begs another question, "What is the CAUSE of this universal intelligence that is CAUSE of the organizing principle?" Chiropractic does NOT address this question. It is beyond the realm of chiropractic philosophy, science, and art. "WHY" you may ask? Because the starting point of **chiropractic's basic science** is the universal principle of organization and the science aspect of chiropractic is the "WHAT" of chiropractic.[1: p.xiv]

Today, given the knowledge of the 2020s, we acknowledge the relationship between cause and effect and between effect and cause. The three aspects of chiropractic, namely, philosophy, science, and art, are separate and distinct from each other, yet these three aspects are absolutely vital to the existence of chiropractic. Chiropractic cannot exist without science (basic and applied), art, and philosophy. The 33 principles of chiropractic's basic science need chiropractic's applied science. We must apply the 33 principles in order to practice the chiropractic objective through the chiropractic art. Chiropractic science (basic and applied) cannot live without chiropractic philosophy; otherwise, it would lead to mindless activism. Chiropractic science and chiropractic philosophy intersect at the innate principles and have mutual synergy. It is also true that chiropractic philosophy needs chiropractic science; otherwise, chiropractic would remain an empty idealism.

As previously stated, in chiropractic, we have overemphasized its philosophy at the very detriment of its science and its art. There is a definite need to integrate the three aspects of chiropractic and to study its "relations between Cause and Effect, and Effect and Cause".[1: p.256] This relationship between cause and effect may be expressed in the formula: if A is the cause of B and B is the cause of C, then A may also be regarded as the cause of C. In fact, the cause survives in its effect. An important characteristic of the relationship between cause and effect is its **CONTINUAL** connection. Its chain has neither beginning nor end (pri. 1). It is never broken; it extends **continually** from one link to another. Its internal mechanism is associated with the instructive information/F expressed by E/matter and manifested as motion (pri. 13, 14). It operates **everywhere** there is existence (pri. 1); therefore it is universal.

In the chiropractic science context, the universal principle of organization continually supplies instructive information/F to all E/matter causing the unification of the three necessary **united** factors, namely, the organizing principle, information/F, and E/matter (pri. 3, 4). This **hard to vary,** explanation of the relationship between cause and effect leads through deductive reasoning to the logical and rational conclusion of the chiropractic objective, namely, the correction of vertebral subluxation for the restoration of TRANSMISSION of conducted innate information/F. The study of the 33 principles of chiropractic's basic science has ALWAYS been known to be about "the relations between Cause and Effect, and Effect and Cause".[1: p.256]

Re-contextualized, principle #17 states:

No. 17. CAUSE AND EFFECT.

EVERY EFFECT HAS A CAUSE AND EVERY CAUSE HAS EFFECTS.

LIVING E/MATTER

18

No. 18. Evidence of Life. The signs of life are evidence of the intelligence of life.

In the 1920s, Stephenson introduced the innate principles explaining that E/matter demonstrates more complex levels of organization that give rise to living E/matter. This type of organization differs from non-living E/matter due to the adaptability of information/F causing E/matter to live and to adapt. These different levels of organization are "motions of the adaptive kind which show the presence and government of a localized intelligence".[1: p.256] Recall that it really is the same organizing principle at work. "The same chemical elements are found in both, the animate and the inanimate.[21: p.3] It is the level of organization of the structures of E/matter that changes, not the principle.

Today, given the knowledge of the 2020s, we understand that adapted universal instructive information/F causes E/matter to live and to adapt to its internal and external environments demonstrating observable levels of organization that are more complex. The motions of living E/matter manifest behaviors within intrinsic limitations (pri. 24), called signs of life. We have identified five specific signs of living E/matter. They are namely, assimilation, excretion, adaptability, growth, and reproduction. Not all these signs need to be present for a living thing to be considered alive. Only one sign needs to be present. These more complex levels of organization are governed by the organizing principle in a NEW way that is capable of processing, coding, and adapting information/F into instructions for E/matter to demonstrate one or more signs of life. This implies well-defined computations, from an essential extension of a universal organizing principle that is intrinsic to living E/matter, that are adapting instructive information/F and E/matter maintaining it alive (pri. 21) ONLY **if it is possible** according to universal laws and for a limited time only, which is the life span of the living thing (pri. 24).

In the chiropractic science context, we witness the emergence of a NEW way that the organizing principle works. It functions as informed dynamics of different motions giving rise to living things. The motions involved in living systems span the broadest outlook from non-living E/matter to adaptive living E/matter up the ladder of complexity demonstrating the ability to respond to a stimulus. These different states of molecular organization are carbon-based and include, the DNA, RNA, proteins, and metabolite levels.

Re-contextualized, principle #18 states:

No. 18. EVIDENCE OF LIFE.

THE SIGNS OF LIFE ARE EVIDENCE OF THE ADAPTIVE ORGANIZATION OF LIFE.

19

No. 19. Organic Matter. The material of the body of a "living thing" is organized matter.

In the 1920s, Stephenson saw the relationship between different levels of "structures of molecules and atoms, which have been assembled for the purpose of functioning adaptively".[1: p.256] The organic E/matter of living things has a sign of life called adaptability. This literally means that is adaptable.

Today, with the knowledge of the 2020s, we realize that at every increasing level of complexity of E/matter, novel features of organization emerge that do not exist at previously observed lower levels of complexity. All E/matter is organized (inorganic and organic), however living E/matter reacts differently. Living things have the ability to RESPOND to stimulus. It is important to differentiate this unique characteristic of living E/matter. It is organized in a way that is uniquely different than non-living E/matter. This uniqueness rests with the fact of the ability of E/matter to be adaptable and can be constructed into the body of a living thing.

Within the chiropractic science context, all E/matter is organized. However, living E/matter is animated and reacts differently due to its ability to be adapted by the essential extension of the organizing principle, the innate law (pri. 23), and in turn to be able to adapt its internal and external environment. The deliberate conversion in character of instructive information/F, that has been computed, coded, and adapted in a NEW way by the organizing principle is applied in the transformation paradigm of E/matter from non-living to living. E/matter moves from condensed E/matter to more and more highly organized E/matter into living E/matter manifesting the five signs of life. This reveals a definite conversion in character of instructive information/F introducing the law that animates E/matter, namely the innate law of living things, which is an essential extension of the universal principle of organization. It also implies a **relationship** of parts working in coordination (pri. 23, 32) within living things. Therefore, living E/matter is organized into a more complex animate state.

Re-contextualized, principle #19 states:

No. 19. ORGANIC E/MATTER.

THE MATERIAL OF THE BODY OF A LIVING THING IS ORGANIC E/MATTER.

WHAT--- HOW--- WHY

At principle #18, Stephenson introduced principles that animate the body of living things; they require a greater understanding of the three aspects of chiropractic, namely, that of science, art, and philosophy, as being SEPARATE and DISTINCT from each other. Chiropractic's applied science aims at truths regarding vertebrates; it applies the principles of chiropractic's basic science, as a solid foundational platform to construct a profession that practices its rational and logical concluded objective. Chiropractic aims to apply its principles to practice chiropractic for **"WHAT"** it is, based on its own **science.** Chiropractic **art** makes specific use of the application of the principles of chiropractic's basic science in practice. Art is the practice of **"HOW"** chiropractic does what it does. Then there is chiropractic **philosophy,** which is concerned with all the assumptions, foundations, methods, and implications of chiropractic's basic science for the use and merit of chiropractic's applied science. **"WHY** chiropractic does what it does".[1: p.vii]

Chiropractic uses mostly rational logic and deductive reasoning in order to formulate specific truths from a general truth, namely principle #1, the universal principle of organization. Principle #1 is the starting point of chiropractic's basic science and is appropriated by chiropractors, as the meaning of existence (pri. 2). The universal principle of organization is to chiropractic what "1+1=2" is to mathematics. Therefore, principle #1 is ABSOLUTE, DUPLICABLE, AND CONSTANT.

From this point, you use deductive reasoning and rational logic to elaborate on the outcomes, meanings, and manifestations of this one general and basic truth.

There is a need to stress the requirement that observations made for the purpose of formulating the principles of chiropractic's basic science include ALL of E/matter with ALL of its intrinsic instructive information/F governed by a universal principle of organization. For this reason, we must understand that chiropractic's basic science is the bedrock of its foundational platform that gives rise to its structural form revealing the chiropractic objective. Science, however, is restricted to those areas where there is general agreement on the nature of the observations involved. It is comparatively easy to agree on observations of physical phenomena, harder to agree on observation of metaphysical phenomena, and difficult in the extreme to reach agreement on matters of theology (and thus the latter remains outside the purview of chiropractic).

So far, we have **re-contextualized** the universal principles and as such, they have led us to NEW observations of more complex levels of organization of E/matter. This ladder of complexity moves from condensed inanimate E/matter that is nonliving, to adaptable animate E/matter that is living. We observe that living E/matter demonstrates patterns of complex organization, as signs of life (pri. 18) that are different from non-living E/matter.

D.D. Palmer wrote, "Chiropractic is a name I originated to designate the science and art of adjusting vertebrae. It does not relate to the study of etiology, or any branch of medicine. Chiropractic includes the science and art of adjusting vertebrae – the know-how and the doing".[4: p.316] He also acknowledged that the non-discrete (non-material) was coupled with the discrete (material), asserting,"The basic principle, and the principles of Chiropractic which have been developed from it, are NOT new. They are as old as the vertebrate. I DO CLAIM, HOWEVER, TO BE THE FIRST TO REPLACE DISPLACED VERTEBRAE BY USING THE SPINOUS AND TRANSVERSE PROCESSES AS LEVERS WHEREWITH TO RACK SUBLUXATED VERTEBRAE INTO NORMAL POSITION, AND FROM THIS BASIC FACT, TO CREATE A SCIENCE WHICH IS DESTINED TO REVOLUTIONALIZE THE THEORY AND PRACTICE OF THE HEALING ART." He also wrote, "The universe is composed of the invisible and visible, spirit and matter. Life is but the expression of spirit thru matter. To make life manifest requires the union of spirit and body."[4: p.527] From these exact quotes of the Founder of chiropractic, we are bound to realize that chiropractic PRACTICALLY relates to living E/matter of the subphylum animal vertebrate; it PHILOSOPHICALLY relates to all other kingdoms of living E/matter; it also SCIENTIFICALLY relates all E/matter since it appropriates the universal principle of organization as its starting point. Interestingly, we also note that it was Isaac Newton, some 200 years before D.D., who is found to contemplate the union of the non-material and the material as he wrote to his friend Richard Bentley,

"The last clause of your second Position I like very well. Tis unconceivable that inanimate brute matter should (without the mediation of something else which is not material) operate upon and affect other matter without mutual contact; as it must if gravitation in the sense of Epicurus be essential and inherent in it. And this is one reason why I desired you would not ascribe innate gravity to me. That gravity should be innate, inherent and essential to matter so that one body may act upon another at a distance through a vacuum without the mediation of anything else, by and through which their action or force may be conveyed from one to another is to me so great an absurdity that I believe no man who has in philosophical matters any

competent faculty of thinking can ever fall into it. Gravity must be caused by an agent acting constantly according to certain laws, but whether this agent be material or immaterial is a question I have left to the consideration of my readers. "[22: p.7]

It is Daniel David Palmer who first postulated this "consideration" of Isaac Newton, and in so doing, constructed a **"SCIENCE WHICH IS DESTINED TO REVOLUTIONALIZE** THE THEORY AND PRACTICE OF THE HEALING ART".[4: p.315]

INTRODUCTION TO THE INNATE
PRINCIPLES OF LIVING E/MATTER

20

No. 20. Innate Intelligence. A "living thing" has an inborn intelligence within its body, called Innate Intelligence.

Let us note that in the 1920s, Stephenson instructed us to see innate intelligence as a "MATHEMATICAL LAW of nature." He wrote, "Let us, in this step of our study, look upon Innate Intelligence less romantically and more scientifically. Not as a little god coldly aloof somewhere in our bodies; who we personify with a capitalized name and whom the more conceited of us think we must chastise occasionally; but a mathematical law of nature."[1: p.257-258] However, Stephenson never really developed this intuitive observation that happens to be true and that is confirmed by chiropractic's basic science today.

The third law of Newton states, "To an action there is always a contrary and equal reaction".[14: p.30] There is always an equalizing balance of actions within E/matter in order to be **maintained** in existence (pri.1). Living E/matter also requires an equalizing balance of information/F (external and internal) in order to be alive. It is a balance between an input of universal information/F within E/matter that is computed, coded, and adapted by a NEW law, and an output that is the expression of adapted E/matter which is manifested as motion that is an equalizing balance in order to maintain living E/matter **alive** (pri. 13, 14). Stephenson wrote, "But there is this difference: in the body, normally, Innate keeps these forces all balanced, controlled, adapted to her uses at all times – every moment".[1: p.267]

Within the chiropractic science context, we can observe a wide range of ever more sophisticated complex properties and actions of E/matter and universal information/F. They demonstrate highly organized manifestations that give rise to the ability of E/matter to be adaptable. As previously stated, we also observe a differentiation of E/matter between non-living and living. Therefore, there is a fundamental and universal scientific organizing principle that is operating at every level of organization to **maintain** E/matter in existence, and sometimes, to maintain it **as living** for a while within its lifespan limitations. This adaptability of E/matter is CAUSED by a NEW law called the **innate law of living things (ILLT).** It is an essential extension of the universal principle of organization to govern living E/matter. This innate law maintains the body of a living thing **alive** within its limitations according to universal laws (pri. 24).

Within these different levels of organization, the essential extension of the organizing principle called the innate law of living things now computes, codes, and adapts universal information/F to construct even more complex organizations of E/matter giving rise to living E/matter. This newly coded information/F transforms and constructs atoms into molecules, molecules into compounds, and compounds into living tissue cells for use in the body. These NEW structural forms of E/matter are constructed and governed by what is now called, the innate law of living things (ILLT). As a result of this NEW adapted universal information/F and E/matter there is a NEW re-formation or re-construction of the structural forms of E/matter that is now manifesting signs of life (pri. 18). This NEW innate law is adding a NEW character to E/matter transforming the properties and actions of E/matter into ACTIVE organization (meaning living E/matter). This NEW adapting, controlling, and balancing law is called the innate law of living things and is intrinsic EXCLUSIVELY to living E/matter. Stephenson wrote, "Universal energies permeate every cell. But there is this difference: in the body, normally, Innate keeps these forces all balanced, controlled, and adapted to her uses all times – every moment".[1: p.267] Therefore, this innate law adapts, and balances universal information/F and E/matter based on principle #1 that **maintains** all E/matter in existence.

For example, E/matter can be added to the body by input of mass flow in the form of food. Since information/F is originally computed to **maintain** E/matter in existence, the usual adapted E/matter balancing the basic representative equation is seen in physiology as: $R = I-E$ where "R" is the rate of kcal that are stored, "I" is the rate of kcal that is ingested and "E" is the rate of kcal expended. This NEW computation is caused by the innate law of living things that is processing, coding, and adapting information/F and E/matter in order to keep E/matter **alive.** The fundamental universal principle of organization of all E/matter essentially extends itself to become specific to the body of a living thing, and gives rise to a different organizational state of E/matter. This NEW reconstruction of the structural forms of E/matter reveals a **RELATIONSHIP** between parts, through interoperability, that are expressing the signs of life. It is this innate law that is responsible for adapting, controlling, and re-constructing (or re-forming) this specific E/matter into the body of a living thing in order to maintains it alive for a while within limits of E/matter and time (pri. 24).

Re-contextualized, principle #20 states:

No. 20. INNATE LAW OF LIVING THINGS.

AN INBORN ORGANIZING PRINCIPLE GOVERNS THE BODY OF A LIVING THING, CALLED THE INNATE LAW OF LIVING THINGS.

WHERE DOES CHIROPRACTIC PHILOSOPHY BEGIN?

At this more complex level of organization of living E/matter, we can easily realize that the demarcation between chiropractic science and chiropractic philosophy is at the core of the nature of chiropractic. Both chiropractic science and chiropractic philosophy need each other. Chiropractic's basic science is useful to chiropractic philosophy and chiropractic philosophy is useful to chiropractic's basic science. Chiropractic's basic science starts with the fundamental universal principle of organization that **maintains** all non-living AND living E/matter in **existence** (pri. 1). D.D. Palmer wrote, "Chiropractic is the name of a classified, indexed knowledge of successive sense impressions of biology—the science of life—which science I created out of principles **which have existed as long as the vertebrate**" (emphasis mine).[14: p.1] Chiropractic philosophy, on the other hand, starts with the innate law of living things that maintains ONLY living E/matter **alive**. (pri. 20). This is due to the fact that CHIROPRACTIC is about, as D.D. Palmer wrote, "TO REPLACE DISPLACED VERTEBRAE BY USING THE SPINOUS AND TRANSVERSE PROCESSES".[4: p.280] Chiropractic philosophy is concerned with "WHY" we apply the principles of its own basic science to the living vertebrates. The innate law of living things is simply the universal principle of organization acting through more complex organizational states of E/matter manifesting motions that pertains exclusively to living E/matter which is distinct from non-living E/matter. [1: p.262] Therefore, chiropractic philosophy starts at principle #20, the innate law of living things, since the purpose of chiropractic is to correct vertebral subluxations, which is found EXCLUSIVELY in the body of living vertebrates. Of course, the previous principles are fundamental to existence and they are operative to EVERYTHING that is **maintained** in existence, including living vertebrates. To reiterate for emphasis, we use chiropractic philosophy when we observe that organization bespeaks intelligence; then we assert that a universal intelligence is the CAUSE of the universal principle of organization. As an example, it is like flying an aircraft. The pilot in command understands that the fundamental principle of the **SCIENCE** of aviation begins with the universal law of gravitation that is acting on a flight from New York to Miami. However, the pilot in command will use aviation's **PHILOSOPHY** with the scientific law of aerodynamics (how air FLOWS around objects) and the laws of flight (airfoil, lift, thrust, drag, power, etc.) in order to explain why they introduce their **ART** in the form of a specific control input to the aircraft for a normal FLOW of air to fly the aircraft on course (aviation's objective). The universal law of gravitation is intrinsic to their flight no matter what, and the fact that they know and understand it, is sufficient. It is the same thing with a chiropractor in their practice as they understands that the fundamental principles of the **SCIENCE** of chiropractic begins with the universal principle of organization that is **maintaining** all E/matter in existence; however, they will use chiropractic **PHILOSOPHY** with the scientific innate law of living things (how E/matter and universal information/F are adapted and FLOWS through the nerve system of vertebrates) and the principles of locating, analyzing and correcting vertebral subluxations (analysis and adjusting techniques) in order to explain "WHY" they introduces their **ART** in the form of a specific adjustic thrust input for a normal FLOW of innate impulses to restore its normal "on course" transmission (chiropractic's objective). The universal principle of organization is intrinsic to their practice no matter what, and the fact that they know and understands it, is sufficient. (By the way, also intrinsic to the practice of chiropractic, are the universal laws of gravitation and of motion, even though we never really think of it this way. It is as intrinsic as the universal principle of organization and the innate law of living things are to piloting an aircraft, even though we never really think of it this way). In both instances, aviation **SCIENCE** and chiropractic **SCIENCE** start at their initial principles, namely, universal gravitation and universal organization. However, both aviation **PHILOSOPHY** and chiropractic **PHILOSOPHY,** start at their useful practical principles, the law of aerodynamics and the innate law of living things.

This starting point of chiropractic philosophy reveals a common denominator in all expressions of life. By using the innate law as the starting point of chiropractic philosophy, it is congruent with D.D. Palmer when he stated, **"I DO CLAIM, HOWEVER, TO BE THE FIRST** TO REPLACE DISPLACED VERTEBRAE BY USING THE SPINOUS AND TRANSVERSE PROCESSES AS LEVERS WHEREWITH TO RACK SUBLUXATED VERTEBRAE INTO NORMAL POSITION, AND FROM THIS BASIC FACT, --- **TO CREATE A SCIENCE** --- WHICH IS **DESTINED TO REVOLUTIONALIZE** THE THEORY AND PRACTICE OF THE HEALING ART." (emphasis mine)[4: p.904]

Chiropractic philosophy is the foundation of our orientations using mostly the principles of living E/matter that are part of chiropractic's basic science. Chiropractic philosophy explains the application (chiropractic's applied science) of some particular principles in order to practice the chiropractic objective. Chiropractors may always use the initial principles of all

E/matter (living and non-living) comprising chiropractic's basic science to develop a greater understanding of the genesis of the chiropractic meaning of existence (pri. 2). Chiropractic science and chiropractic philosophy need each other so that chiropractors can develop an explanation that is **hard to vary** in order to demonstrate the **universal** values of chiropractic to the public.

It is clear that, principle #1 through principle #17 are the initial fundamental and universal principles of chiropractic's basic science constructing the foundational platform of the "WHAT" chiropractic is. The first principle is the initial CAUSE of organization supplying properties and action that **maintain** all E/matter in existence (pri. 1). Of course, **maintaining** E/matter in existence will always be a time dependent process (pri. 6). The function of universal information/F will always be to **unite** the non-discrete, non-physical organizing principle with the discrete, physical material E/matter (pri. 10). All E/matter will always express information/F (pri. 13) and manifest it as motion (pri. 14). Every effect will always have a cause and every cause will always have effects (pri. 17). Then after the initial principles, we encounter the **innate principles** that are the fundamental basis of **living things** continuing the genesis of chiropractic's basic science; these innate principles are included in the nature of the "WHAT" of chiropractic. After all, chiropractic philosophy will always be the "WHY" of chiropractic. It explains very clearly "WHY" chiropractic does "WHAT" it does, and "HOW" it does it. Therefore, chiropractic philosophy truly start with the fundamental principle #20, the innate law of living things.

21

No. 21. The Mission of Innate Intelligence. The mission of Innate Intelligence is to maintain the material of the body of a "living thing" in active organization.

In the 1920s, inasmuch as he instructed us to look at innate intelligence as "mathematical law of nature", Stephenson personified this scientific innate law of living things (ILLT) and assigned to it some anthropomorphic attributes. The originator of this antropomorphism is D.D. Palmer himself as he wrote, on 'Innate Intelligence' that he was the originator of every idea in Chiropractic up to the time he left Davenport. B.J. Palmer, throughout the Green Books, passionately used the pronoun "she" referring to this innate law. B.J. also referred to the afferent side of the Nine Primary Functions as "The Wife".[1: p.189] Once again, we must remember that the educated intelligence of our predecessors was individually and collectively developing according to the knowledge and context of their era. Today, our individual and collective educated intelligence continues to develop according the knowledge and context of our era. Later, the educated intelligence of future generations will CONTINUALLY develop according to the knowledge and context of their era. The capability of our educated brain to function is truly a prisoner of its own time, for better or for worse.

The word mission comes from a Latin word that means, "to send" or "a specific task with which a *person or group* is charged". As we can see, the word "mission" does not describe what the purpose of something is. Mission is ascribed to people. On the other hand, a purpose according to the Merriam-Webster dictionary is an end to be attained. It is the reason why something exists. Since D.D. and B.J. anthropomorphized "Innate", principle #21 mentioned that "she" (innate), has a mission. Mission is about people. However, scientific principles do not have a mission, they have a purpose, an end to be attained.

According to principle #5 of chiropractic's basic science, and the laws of conservation, the universe is complete. First, there are properties and actions supplied to all E/matter (non-living and living) from the universal principle of organization that **maintains** it in existence (pri. 1). From principle #1, we recognize that the universal principle of organization continually supplies instructive information/F to the body of a living thing to **maintain** its living E/matter in existence. This instructive information/F from the organizing principle is, in turn, computed, coded, and adapted into innate information/F, by the innate law of living things to maintain the body **alive** within the limitations of E/matter (pri. 24).

Within the chiropractic science context, the living body is by nature comprised of dynamic chemistry due to the innate law of living things continually computing, coding, and adapting innate information/F into instruction features. This innate law is, moment-to-moment, a 100%/perfect software capable of computing, coding, and adapting information/F into instructions that maintain the E/matter of the body **alive,** within its limitations. The **purpose** of this innate law to keep the body *alive, if it is possible,* according to universal laws (pri. 24). Stephenson puts it this way, "This force or message is specific for the momentary needs of a tissue cell. It must therefore be a more highly organized force than that given to molecules and atoms".[1: p.265]

Re-contextualized, principle #21 states:

No. 21. THE PURPOSE OF THE INNATE LAW OF LIVING THINGS.

THE PURPOSE OF THE INNATE LAW OF LIVING THINGS IS TO MAINTAIN THE MATERIAL OF THE BODY OF A LIVING THING ALIVE.

22

No. 22. The Amount of Innate Intelligence. There is 100% of Innate Intelligence in every "living thing," the requisite amount, proportional to its organization.

In the 1920s, Stephenson specifies principle #22 as being "The Quality of Innate Intelligence," yet he wrote that innate intelligence "the 'Quantity' of Innate Intelligence in one thing *may* not be as much as the "Quantity" in another living thing, but it is the requisite amount, hence one hundred percent for that thing".[1: p.261] Stephenson mentioned that "Degree in Chiropractic terminology is taken to mean 'degree of perfection;' therefore, it involves quality as well as quantity"[1: p.240,261] He seems to infer that a living thing may not have as much innate law (innate intelligence) as another but that it is "the requisite amount *proportional* for each." Of course, it is not possible to quantify a non-discrete (non-physical) entity because it cannot be divided into parts since it is non-material. There cannot be a measurement of a non-physical entity according to principle #7. It is always 100% perfect (i.e., the amount of organization for any particle of E/matter is always 100%/perfect). As an example, the universal principle of gravity of planet earth is 100% perfect for every particle of E/matter on planet earth; gravity can be used to work with the principle of aerodynamics in order for E/matter to be airborne. Yet, gravity is always 100% perfect regardless of the quality or quantity of E/matter.

Today, with the knowledge of the 2020s, we now understand that the innate law is always acting 100%/perfect in every living cells of living E/matter regardless of their properties or actions. This innate law of living things is 100%/perfect for ALL living E/matter regardless of the complexity of its organization. There is 100%/perfect organization at the living cell level, at the living organ level, at the living system level and also at the whole living body level within the limitation of E/matter (pri. 24). This means that every adaptive process of living E/matter is ALWAYS perfect within its limitations any given moment. There is an integral innate processing for continual adaptation moment to moment that is ALWAYS 100%/perfect.

Re-contextualized, principle #22 states:

No. 22. THE QUALITY OF THE INNATE LAW OF LIVING THINGS.

THE INNATE LAW OF LIVING THINGS IS ALWAYS 100%/ PERFECT FOR ALL LIVING E/MATTER.

23

No. 23. The Function of Innate Intelligence. The function of Innate Intelligence is to adapt universal forces and matter for use in the body, so that all parts of the body will have coordinated action for mutual benefit.

In the 1920s Stephenson wrote, "Innate Intelligence, the law of organization, continually coordinates the forces and material within the organism to keep it actively organized... **it is scientifically speaking, the principle of organization**".[1: p.262] As we continue to re-contextualize the principles of chiropractic's basic science, we realize that the innate law, re-organizes, computes, and adapts universal information/F into NEW instructive codes that maintains E/matter alive. This "investing with NEW character" of information/F and E/matter adapts it for use in the body thereby maintaining the body **alive** through coordinated action of all its parts according to universal laws (pri. 24). Stephenson also wrote, "Then Innate Intelligence is the coordinating principle".[1: p.332]

Today, with the knowledge of the 2020s, we recognize that the ability of E/matter to undergo continual cellular differentiation, reproduction, and replacement is through adaptive re-organization that is comprised of deconstruction and reconstruction (pri. 26), generating a dynamic chemistry controlled by the innate law of living things.

Within the chiropractic science context, the innate law computes, codes, and adapts universal information/F and E/matter investing it "with NEW character" for use in the body. This ACT of computing, coding, and adapting is the function of the innate law of living things. This investing "with NEW character" actually controls and governs all the tissue cells, and coordinates the actions of all the parts of the body for mutual benefit within the limitations of E/matter and time (pri. 24).

Re-contextualized, principle #23 states;

No. 23. THE FUNCTION OF THE INNATE LAW OF LIVING THINGS.

THE FUNCTION OF THE INNATE LAW OF LIVING THINGS IS TO ADAPT UNIVERSAL INFORMATION/F AND E/MATTER FOR USE IN THE BODY, SO THAT ALL PARTS OF THE BODY WILL HAVE COORDINATED ACTION FOR MUTUAL BENEFIT.

24

No. 24. The Limits of Adaptation. Innate Intelligence adapts forces and matter for the body as long as it can do so without breaking a universal law, or Innate Intelligence is limited by the limitations of matter.

In the 1920s Stephenson's concept of limitations of matter is understood from the point of view "that extreme adaptation cannot be made for the body"[1; p.263] In those days, Cricks and Watson had not yet discovered the double helix structure of the DNA containing the encoded genetic information of all living things. Today, we know that the limitation of living E/matter is due in part to the laws of genetics intrinsic to the DNA. For example, the genetic characteristics of a polar bear will not sustain 110°F, yet it will be comfortable at -50°F. A panther, on the other hand, will die quickly at -50°F, but it will be comfortable at 110°F. Each species has its own genetic characteristics regarding the capability of its E/matter to be adapted. It is a universal law of genetics. Natural longevity and life span are also included within this genetic law. Intrinsic to the limitations of living E/matter, contained within its DNA, is a generative motion that is limited by time. All living E/matter has a "life-time-limit" intrinsic to its nature. It is information/F and E/matter adapted by the innate law that is maintaining the body of living things **alive** (pri. 20, 21, 22). It is the "shelf life" of the power supply components, generating living motion to the body in order for E/matter to be **as living.** Ultimately, the body of a living thing has an expiration date that the innate law of living things will comply with and will not break (pri. 24). The longevity of living things has its own specific limits with regards to living E/matter depending on its genetic code contained within the double helix of its DNA. Of course, the limitations of E/matter that B. J. and Stephenson intuitively understood in the 1920s still hold true today and is now confirmed by the knowledge of the 2020s.

Today, with the knowledge of the 2020s, we realize that the equation $E=mc^2$ is based on energy transfer, that E/matter undergoes deconstruction and reconstruction processes (pri. 26). These are instructed dynamics from the universal principle of organization that **maintains** E/matter in existence. Regarding living E/matter, these processes are adapted by the innate law of living things only according to *what is possible* from universal laws (pri. 24). This inborn adaptive law will not break a universal law. That is due to the limitations of living E/matter. Chiropractic has a solid foundational platform based on universal principles of *what is possible* **ALL THE TIME.**

Within the chiropractic science context, the innate law of living things will adapt information/F and E/matter within the limit of adaptation of living E/matter. This limitation of living E/matter is dependent upon **what is possible** in terms of the E/matter's adaptability according to universal laws and the interactive **relationship** between these laws. It is not possible for anything to break a universal law due to its universality. Therefore, the innate law of living things will not break a universal law, be it gravity, motion, action/reaction, conservation of E/matter, genetics, limitation of E/matter etc... Stephenson wrote, "None but the Creator can change a law, make laws, or circumvent physical laws, so the life current must be a force directly from Law itself."[1 p.264] This direct quote underscores that neither intelligence nor the organizing principle are the creator. Intelligence and the organizing principle are limited by the limitation of E/matter and will NOT break a universal law (pri. 24). The limitation of time is intrinsic to principle #24. For example, the digestion of a meal requires time. If you were to eat food before the previous digestion is completed, you might vomit because it requires more time for your body to digest the previous meal (pri. 6). The innate law of living thing is limited by the limitations of living E/matter and time.

Re-contextualized, principle #24 states:

No. 24. THE LIMITS OF ADAPTATION.

THE INNATE LAW OF LIVING THINGS ADAPTS INFORMATION/F AND E/MATTER FOR THE BODY ONLY IF IT IS POSSIBLE ACCORDING TO UNIVERSAL LAWS.

25

No. 25. The Character of Innate Forces. The forces of Innate Intelligence never injure or destroy the structures in which they work.

In the 1920s, Stephenson wrote, "This life shows that it is an adaptable law, able to make *instantaneous* changes according to environmental conditions of a tissue cell".[1: p.264]

Today with the knowledge of the 2020s, we now understand that the universe is an entity made of physical and nonphysical, material and non-material, discrete and non-discrete aspects. Since there is a whole lot more empty space than there is E/matter, it is fact that E/matter is contained WITHIN space-time. The material is within the non-material and the non-material is also within the material. Remember that it was Einstein who was further developing Newton's view of time "flowing uniformly" and called 'duration by means of motion' ."[14: p.23] It must be noted that E/matter is **maintained** in existence as a result of its properties and actions being supplied by the universal principle of organization, from its organizing information/F that unites E/matter with the organizing principle. All E/matter has motion (pri. 14) demonstrating that the configuration of electrons, protons, and neutrons, AND their velocities are **intrinsic** to all space and time. The motions of the particles of E/matter cover distance within space that can be measured and quantified in time (pri. 6). It is becoming clear that, as Stephenson mentioned, "Time is an element necessary to the bond between intelligence and matter."[1: p.239] This reveals a new equation in the form of, E/matter = Space/time. The "E" and the "m" of $E=mc^2$ are now just items to go on one side of the "=" sign linking them.[9: p.206] Therefore, within the EXISTENCE of our universe, there is a bond between the material and the non-material. It is information/F (pri. 10), and its mathematical sign within the equation is the " = " sign. It is the "missing link." The equation for existence is: universal principle of organization = E/matter. The "=" is the organized information/F which is the bond that **unites** the non-material organizing principle and the material E/matter.

Within the chiropractic science context, we now understand that the innate law of living thing is 100%/perfect intrinsic in ALL living things (pri. 20). It adapts universal information/F and E/matter **ONLY IF IT IS POSSIBLE** ACCORDING TO UNIVERSAL LAWS (pri. 24). This innate law brings about specific adjustments through adaptation in order to make error correction under innate dynamics that are balancing information/F within limitation of E/matter. These specific adjustments maintain the adaptability of the body. These adjustments are, in fact, error corrections that facilitate the reconstruction of living E/matter for coordination of action (pri. 32) and are congruent with keeping the body of the living thing **alive** (pri. 21).

It is the innate law that adapts information/F and E/matter investing them with a NEW character facilitating the dynamics of error correction for coordination of action of all the parts of the body for mutual benefit (pri. 23). The result is *instantaneous* constructive interactive relationships with the internal and external environment of the tissue cell, moment to moment. Innate information/F is coordinated instruction dynamics that ALWAYS re-construct and NEVER de-construct the structure of E/matter within the limits of adaptation (pri. 24). It is when the limitations of the body's E/matter have been fully or completely reached at a specific moment in time, that the E/matter of the body is no longer adaptable for coordination of action and death ensues. It is then that the unadapted universal information/F will deconstruct the structures of E/matter to its most basic state (molecules and atoms).

We observe that the innate information/F is the dynamic instruction expressed by the tissue cells, which are manifesting motion as the signs of life (pri.13, 14, 18). Stephenson calls these dynamic innate instructions "mental force" and he wrote, "This force or message is specific for the momentary needs of a tissue cell. It must therefore be a more highly organized force than that given to molecules and atoms."[1: p.265] This means that the innate law of living things is CONTINUALLY computing, encoding, and adapting information/F and E/matter, **as long as it is possible,** in accordance with universal laws for the welfare of the body (pri. 23, 24). The innate law of living things is 100%/perfecft and its function is 100%/perfect moment to moment (pri. 22).

The innate law adapts universal information/F and E/matter so that the body manifests motion as the signs of life (pri. 14, 18, 23). When the signs of life are manifested, the innate law (pri. 20) becomes the fundamental principle, and the bedrock of chiropractic practice. As D.D. Palmer wrote, "Chiropractic is a name I originated to designate the science and art of adjusting vertebrae. It does not relate to the study of etiology, or any branch of medicine. Chiropractic includes the science and art of adjusting vertebrae – the know-how and the doing".[4: p.316] It is crystal clear then, that the innate law is a fundamental principle of chiropractic's basic science. This principle is applied by chiropractors for chiropractic's applied science to practice of the chiropractic objective. The aim of which is to correct vertebral subluxations to remove the interference to the transmission of conducted innate information/F (pri. 29, 31). This restores control over the structural and dynamic features of living E/matter with its ever more complex state of organization through coordination of action for mutual benefit. It is the body of the living thing striving to stay alive (pri. 21, 23).

Re-contextualized principle, #25 states;

No. 25. THE CHARACTER OF INNATE INFORMATION/F.

THE INFORMATION/F OF THE INNATE LAW OF LIVING THINGS NEVER INJURES OR DE-CONSTRUCTS THE STRUCTURES IN WHICH IT WORKS.

26

No. 26. Comparison of Universal and Innate Forces. In order to carry on the universal cycle of life, Universal forces are destructive, and Innate forces constructive, as regards structural matter.

In the 1920s Stephenson wrote, "Perhaps some of these energies are not known to us in physics. What right have we to assume that we found them all." He wrote further, "We observe, that energy seems to travel... by radiation and conduction." He also wrote that, "universal intelligence with its universal energies *fills* all the space in the universe, and every spot." (emphasis mine)[1: p. 265-269]

Today, with the knowledge of the 2020s, we know that $E=mc^2$. We have established that force cannot be energy. Force, in chiropractic, is information/F, whether universal or innate. Universal information/F **unites** E/matter and the organizing principle (pri. 10) with strong and weak bonds. At the sub-atomic level, information/F is then expressed by E/matter (pri. 13) and manifested as motion (pri. 14). This is how E/matter is being **maintained** in existence (pri. 1). The level of organization of the atom is the most basic level, and according to Strauss, "...The most intelligent organization of matter is in its simplest atomic form, hence universal intelligence tends to break down matter to that level. Innate intelligence, on the other hand, tends to build up matter to more complex forms that are capable of renewing or restructuring themselves. This is an essential difference between universal and innate intelligence."[13: p. 444]

Fundamental to the atom are the electron, proton, and neutron that are instructed by information/F **uniting** E/matter to the organizing principle **maintaining** existence (pri. 1, 10). Should living E/matter reach its full limits of adaptation (death), then according to Stephenson, "... the living organisms revert to the elemental state wherein their molecules act according to the unswerving laws of physics and chemistry. A living organism has signs of life, which is evidence that it is under the care of intelligence; evidence of special care".[1: p.268] This is understandable since the innate law functions ONLY with **what is possible** according to universal laws (pri. 24).

Within the chiropractic science context, we see that, in the living body, organization exists at the cell level, organ level, system level, and whole body level. Therefore, the innate information/F is both radiated and conducted within the body of the living thing. Radiated information/F is necessary to control components of the cell for its metabolism (pri. 21). Conducted information/F is necessary for the coordinated actions of all body parts for mutual benefit (pri. 23). This introduces the innate impulse, which is a computed, coded, and adapted conducted information/F for coordination of actions. (The same process takes place for radiated information/F for the innate ray or wave for metabolism). Stephenson says that it is a, "Mental force, that which flows over nerves to their peripheral ending. This force or message is specific for the momentary needs of a tissue cell".[1: p.265] It is a specific computed message that is coded and assembled within the innate field (brain) to be radiated for metabolism of the cells of the body (pri. 21) or conducted through the nerve system for coordination of action of the parts of the body (pri. 23). It is quite easy to understand coordination of action of all the parts of an organism for mutual benefit (pri. 23, 32). However, regarding metabolism it is a little more difficult, although easier to understand with an example. When a heart is transported in a special solution from New York to California for a surgical heart-transplant, the heart continues to function metabolically under the control of the innate law governing the cells of the heart as an organ. The innate information/F is innate rays that are radiated within the heart cells to keep it "alive" until the surgical heart-transplant is performed. Chiropractic does NOT address interference with the radiation of innate rays. Chiropractic addresses **EXCLUSIVELY** one specific type of interference; that of conducted innate impulses that are transmitted through specialized E/matter, the nervous system. This specific interference of transmission of conducted innate information/F is always directly or indirectly caused by what is called the vertebral subluxation (pri. 31). Universal information/F is ALWAYS deconstructive toward structural E/matter (p. 12). However, when it is computed, coded, and adapted by the innate law into an innate information/F it becomes an innate impulse. The innate impulse is innate information/F that is ALWAYS constructive toward structural E/matter (pri. 25). It is an instruction that coordinates the actions of all the parts of the body for mutual benefit (pri. 23). Once again, energy and matter are interchangeable, hence the term, E/matter. Force, in chiropractic, is information, hence the term, information/F. Both, E/matter and information/F, are NEVER created nor destroyed in accordance with principle #1 and the laws of conservation. Therefore, it is appropriate to use the term deconstructive instead of destructive.

Re-contextualized, principle #26 states:

No. 26. COMPARISON OF UNIVERSAL INFORMATION/F AND INNATE INFORMATION/F.

IN ORDER TO CARRY ON THE UNIVERSAL CYCLE OF LIFE, UNIVERSAL INFORMATION/F IS DE-CONSTRUCTIVE, AND INNATE INFORMATION/F IS CONSTRUCTIVE, AS REGARDS STRUCTURAL E/MATTER.

27

No. 27. The Normality of Innate Intelligence. Innate Intelligence is always normal and its function is always normal.

In the 1920s, Stephenson wrote, " Intelligence is always perfect – always one hundred per cent. The forces it assembles are always correct".[1: p.269] According to Merriam-Webster, a principle is "a general or basic truth on which other truths or theories can be based." Our lexicon defines it, "A principle is a fundamental truth that serves as the foundation universal laws." Therefore, the universal principle of organization is the fundamental explanation of scientific laws. The symbolic representation of the universal principle of organization is, $R_1 + R_2 \Delta E = P$. This formula, describing the universal principle of organization, clearly explains that E/matter is never created nor destroyed. It explains the laws of motion, action/reaction, etc.... It is always 100%/perfect, since it **maintains** the material of the universe, (E/matter) in existence (pri. 1). The evidence of more complex organization of E/matter reveals the innate law of living things (pri. 20, 21, 22, 23) that functions with **what is possible** according to universal laws (pri. 24). The innate law is also 100%/perfect for all living E/matter (pri. 22). Its function is, 100%/perfect as well. The innate information/F that has been computed, codified, and adapted is always exact. It is due to the limitation of E/matter (pri. 24) that the message cannot be decoded into the computed instructions of the innate information/F at the body part receptor. It is either because the conducting E/matter is lacking ease, or the receptor body part is not sound. Either way, the imperfection is within the STRUCTURE of E/matter and not within the innate law or its instructive information/F. They are non-discrete and ALWAYS 100%/perfect. With respect to the innate impulse for coordination of action, the interference in transmission is within the conductor nerve cell. The interference occurs between physical brain cell and physical tissue cell. This is extremely important to understand as it explains "WHY" the chiropractic objective is at CAUSE and not effect. For example, say that the instruction of the innate impulse is NOT decoded properly by the receptor body part due to a genetic defect or an injury within the body part itself. There might very well be no subluxation present, and the body part will continue to malfunction. This underscores the limits of adaptation, whereas the function of the innate law is ONLY about **what is possible** according to universal laws (pri. 24).

Within the chiropractic science context, biologically speaking, the adaptation of information/F and E/matter of living things requires specific computation and interactional coded instructive information/F to transmit the innate impulse (message) for specific coordination of action moment to moment. As Stephenson wrote, "This force or message is specific for the momentary needs of a tissue cell".[1: p.265] Moment to moment adaptation is necessary for coordination of activities. The implementation of this instructive information/F for living E/matter is necessary and 100%/perfect normal for the operation of the processor-hardware of the living part for coordination of actions (pri. 32). As it is a time dependent process (pri. 6), E/matter is the only factor of the triune that is discrete and that can be imperfect in its *structural forms,* the other two factors being 100%/ perfect and non-discrete. It is called innate normal. Normality, in chiropractic, is referenced from the point of view of the innate law of living things and its function (pri. 23, 25). It is the CAUSE factor that governs living systems to maintain them **alive** within their limitations (pri. 24). Innate normal is specific to the life of the body moment to moment. In order for E/matter to normally express innate information/F (pri. 13), there must be no interference in the transmitter cells (nerve cells) for the proper conduction of innate impulses, and there must also be no interference of the radiation of innate rays for proper soundness of the tissue of the body part. Chiropractic addresses **ONLY** the transmission of conducted innate impulses.

Re-contextualized, principle #27 states:

No. 27. THE NORMALITY OF THE INNATE LAW OF LIVING THINGS.

THE INNATE LAW OF LIVING THINGS IS ALWAYS NORMAL AND ITS FUNCTION IS ALWAYS NORMAL.

28

No. 28. The Conductors of Innate Forces. The forces of Innate Intelligence operate through or over the nervous system in animal bodies.

In the 1920s, Stephenson wrote, "**The chiropractor aims only to restore** – to bring about restoration. He adds no more current but removes the obstacles to the normal flow *(momentum)* of that which should be supplied to the tissue from the inside."[1: p.270] His understanding of the nervous system is sufficient to elaborate about coordination of action. However, he runs into a problem, due to the use of anthropomorphic qualities regarding the controlling factor of the body. He wrote, "The brain is the headquarters of Innate's control, the seat of the mind".[1: p.271] According to article 43 of the *Chiropractic Text Book*, this statement is not accurate. It is the non-discrete innate brain (field) with a *theoretical location* that is the headquarters of innate intelligence, not the discrete physical brain. The innate field is wherever the innate law is in the body. The innate law is EVERYWHERE in the body. We have already differentiated the innate law of the cell from the innate law of the organ from the innate law of the system, and from the innate law of the body. Therefore, the operating system, that is the headquarters of the innate law, is the innate field (brain) which is EVERYWHERE in the body.[1: p.13]

Today with the knowledge of the 2020s, we understand that the function of the innate law continues to adapt living E/matter into complex organization through coordinated interoperability. The path for keeping E/matter alive covers a full range of innate computation and processes that determine the internal adaptation as well as its interaction with the environment. Indeed the most complex system available is the nerve system; it is innately adapted, wired, integrated, and interconnected with all the parts of the body for coordination of activities (pri. 23).

Within the chiropractic science context, to implement coordination of action of all body parts through adaptation (pri. 23) requires transmission of conducted innate information/F under the control of the innate law of living things. This transmission of conducted innate information/F and reception by all the body parts offers interoperability of living E/matter, moment to moment within limitations, to make error correction that leads to further adaptation for structural constructive purposes. The nerve system serves the purpose of transmitting conducted innate information/F, called innate impulses, in the vertebrate animal bodies.

NON-MATERIAL REALITIES

At this point, it is necessary to discuss some fundamental understanding, according to what we know today, of non-material realities. First of all, a universal principle of organization is intrinsic to all E/matter (pri. 1). Without it, E/matter would NOT be **maintained** in existence. The universal principle of organization is a fundamental organizing principle, which is the principle of continual existence. The function of the universal principle of organization is to **organize** information/F (pri. 8). This fundamental principle organizes unlimited information/F **maintaining** *all* E/matter in existence. Therefore, living E/matter is also **maintained** in existence by this fundamental principle. The body of a living thing is governed by the innate law of living things, which is maintaining it as living (pri. 20) if it is possible according to universal laws (pri. 24). This innate law has been called, "the law of life," by B.J. Palmer. Its function is to adapt universal information/F, invest it with NEW character, and re-assemble it into innate information/F for ALL the tissue cells. We must remember that the innate law of living things can adapt an unlimited supply of universal information/F. The innate law is a part OF the universal principle of organization, in so far as it is intrinsic to the existence of all living E/matter in the entire universe. The innate law is also a part FROM the universal principle of organization, in so far as it is ONLY localized within the body of living things. The innate law is an essential extension of the universal principle of organization. Basically, the innate law is a localized aspect of the universal principle of organization, and as such, it is "under" the rule, of the initial universal principle. As an example, Newton's third law of equal and opposite reaction is "under" the rule of his second law of acceleration of the law of gravity.[14: p.31] The innate law, which is non-material and maintains the body as living, is an *essential extended continuation* of the universal principle of organization that is also non-material, **maintaining** all E/matter in existence (pri. 1). The universal principle of organization is EVERYWHERE in the universe and the innate law of living things is EVERYWHERE within ALL living E/matter in the universe. The universal principle of organization and the innate law of living things are non-material; they are essentially one and the same. The innate law is simply the universal principle ADAPTING more complex levels and states of E/matter. We differentiate them, as universal principle of organization and innate law of living things, for our own understanding. It is the same way when the law of universal gravitation and the law of geometry are differentiated, when they are truly one and the same. "Einstein's general relativity is a mathematically beautiful *application* of geometric ideas to gravitational physics."[23: p.347]

Before we further study the conductor of innate impulses, we must realize that ALL innate information/F must first be assembled before being conducted through the nervous system or radiated from within the all tissue cell. The innate law of living things functions through an operating system within the body that is called the innate brain (it is literally a field) and is also non-discrete (non-material). It is there that innate information/F is assembled. The innate field (brain) is supplied innate impulses and innate rays directly from the innate law. "It is a vital spot and cannot be diseased. Its existence is actual, but its location is theoretical".[1: p.13] It is located within the body of the living thing, wherever the innate law acts. Stephenson wrote, "There is no transmission of mental impulses from Innate Intelligence to Innate brain field. There is no necessity, Innate being right here. For this reason it always has 100% mental impulses".[1: p. 13]

Since living E/matter is continually supplied innate information/F computed by the innate law in order to keep it alive (pri. 21), the innate field (brain) as an operating system, is used for assembling innate information/F. Some of them will emerge, as innate impulses, in the physical brain for centralization and transmission to effectuate coordination of action through the nervous system as conductor. Others will emerge, as innate rays, from within ALL the cells of the body for controlling cellular components to effectuate metabolism. Again, the innate field (brain) must be non-discrete because it is the "vital spot" of assembly of innate information/F of the innate law which is EVERYWHERE within the body. Therefore, the "headquarters" or "operating system" of the innate law of living things is the innate field (brain), which is EVERYWHERE within the body, and must be wherever the innate law is, which is EVERYWHERE within the LIVING body!

At the precise moment of the coding of the innate information/F by the innate law into innate impulses or innate rays, they are assembled within the innate field for conduction through the nerve system for coordination of actions, or for radiation from within the tissue cell controlling its components for metabolism.

INTER-CONNECTIVITY AND INTEROPERABILITY

Principle #27 states that the function of the innate law is ALWAYS normal and that one of the resulting outputs of that function is coordination of action of all the parts of the body for mutual benefit (pri. 23). To have coordination of action, there must be interconnectivity between ALL the parts in order to manifest mutual benefit of ALL the parts of the body. As the innate law adapts universal information/F and E/matter for coordination of action of all the parts of the body for mutual benefit (pri. 23), the congruency of instructive information/F necessary to coordinate all the parts of the body needs organizational interoperability.

In order to re-contextualized the next principle, principle #28, as a comparison to computer data processing will be utilized to demonstrate the transmission of innate impulses within the nervous system. It will be evidenced that the body is truly a computer governed by the innate law, even though the human being is more than the components of computer software and hardware. The body is the integrated motion system through which WE live our life. It is true that "we cannot give what we do not own"; we cannot not invent outside of us that which does not already exist inside of us. It is always from ABOVE-DOWN-INSIDE-OUT.

The innate law of living things adapts universal information/F and E/matter for use in the body so that all parts will have coordinated action for mutual benefit (pri. 23). The innate law governs the body by computing, coding, and adapting inputs of information/F for metabolic use and coordination of action of all the parts of the body (pri. 23). The parts of the body are a set of agents interacting within a finite (pri. 24) process for mutual benefit. An action loop is one the foundational elements for this coordination principle (pri. 23, 32). The innate impulse as input is transmitted from the physical brain (CPU) through the conducting efferent nerves (transmitters), and returns as impressions of output through the afferent nerves (transmitters) back to the physical brain (CPU) for coordination of actions of the body parts (receptors). Forming the an action loop. Coordination tasks can be delegated through computational processes to manage dependencies of flow and instruction sharing among activities. **(See diagram 1).**

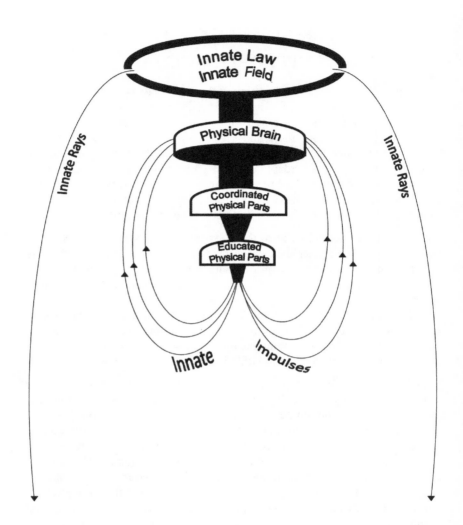

Diagram 1:
Transmission of innate impulses through nerve conduction
from physical brain to physical parts including feedback loop
for coordination of activities, and innate rays through radiation
from within every tissue cell controlling cellular
components for metabolism.

This demonstration of interoperability through interconnectivity will parallel the "Normal Complete Cycle" showing a complex level of organization perpetuated in a cycle (action loop) for coordination of action.[1: p.336] Some terms have been edited or substituted within the Normal Complete Cycle for congruency defined in the lexicon. With regards to the radiation of innate rays this cycle is modified accordingly. However, chiropractic addresses interference in transmission of innate impulses EXCLUSIVELY through correction of subluxation. Chiropractic does not address innate rays.

Edited NORMAL COMPLETE CYCLE, from Stephenson's textbook.[1: p.11]

Universal principle of organization

2- Innate law of living things	30- 100%/perfect instantaneous integral adaptation
3- 100%/perfect innate realm	29- Innate law of living things
4- Brain cell	28- Integral innate processing
5- Innate characterization	27- Sensation/feedback
6- Transformation/coding	26- Interpretation/decoding
7- Innate impulse	25- 100%/perfect processing
8- Propulsion/conductivity	24- Reception
9- Efferent nerve	23- Brain cell
10- Transmission	22- Transmission
11- Tissue cell	21- Afferent nerve
12- Reception	20- Trophic Impulse
13- Physical representation	19- Impression/recoding
14- Expression	18- Vibration
15- Function	17- Tissue cell
16- Coordination	

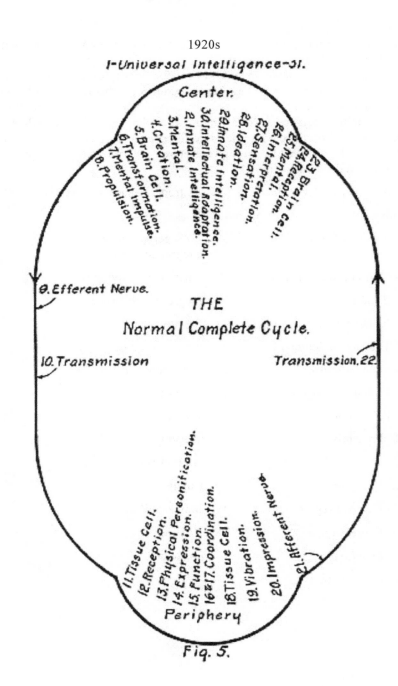

Fig. 5.

2020s
1 - Universal Principle of Organization- 31

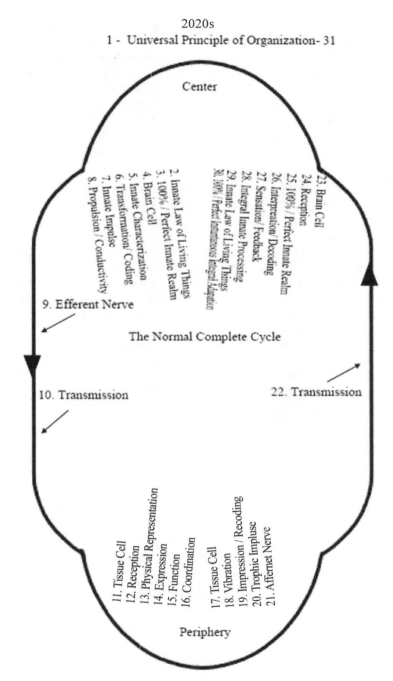

Center

23. Brain Cell
24. Reception
25. 100% / Perfect Innate Realm
26. Interpretation/ Decoding
27. Sensation/ Feedback
28. Integral Innate Processing
29. Innate Law of Living Things
30. 100% / Perfect Instantaneous Integral Adaptive

2. Innate Law of Living Things
3. 100% / Perfect Innate Realm
4. Brain Cell
5. Innate Characterization
6. Transformation/ Coding
7. Innate Impulse
8. Propulsion / Conductivity

9. Efferent Nerve

The Normal Complete Cycle

10. Transmission

22. Transmission

11. Tissue Cell
12. Reception
13. Physical Representation
14. Expression
15. Function
16. Coordination

17. Tissue Cell
18. Vibration
19. Impression / Recoding
20. Trophic Impluse
21. Affernet Nerve

Periphery

From what scientists have learned over the years from data processing, they wrote, "fields programmable gate arrays *(cells, organs, systems, etc...)* consist of a large number of logic block programs *(innate information/F)* that can be configured and reconfigured, individually, to do a wide range of tasks. One logic block may do arithmetic, another signals processing, and yet another look things up in a table. The computation of the whole is a function of how the individual parts are configured. Fields programmable gates arrays *(cells, organs, systems, etc...)* can be reprogrammed to the desired functionality requirements AFTER manufacturing" (emphasis mine).[24]

We now know that the language of neurons and synapses are connected to bodily functions.[25] It appears that the innate law is akin to software (operating system, application programs, coders, device drivers, network interface, etc...). Neurons are akin to computer hardware (CPU, transmitters, hardware platform interface, modulators, processors, microprocessors, decoders, receptors, feedback loop, etc...), and bodily functions are akin to the actions that a computer performs (taking data input, processing instructions, manifesting data output, etc...) The computation of data (information/F) **unites** the software (organizing principle) with the manifestation of data (E/matter) demonstrating the function of information/F (pri. 10). If the heart is a biological pump and the nose is a biological filter, then the physical brain is a biological central processing unit and the nerves are a conductive transmission network system. The nervous system is basically a sophisticated hardware system used to compute and transmit innate information/F, governed by the innate law, for coordination of actions of all the parts of the organism (pri. 23, 32). Here is a model flowchart example that will be applied later *(see diagram 2).*

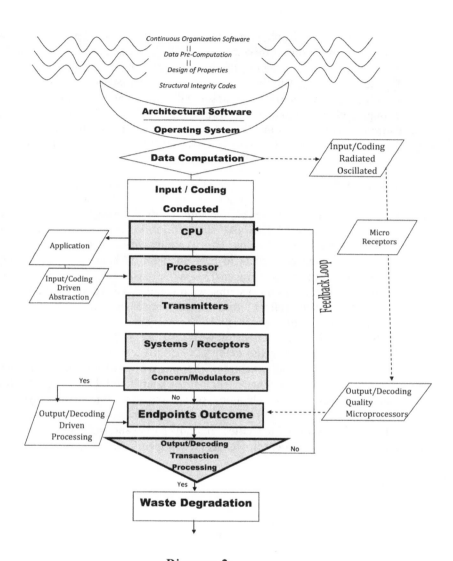

Diagram 2:
Flowchart of the universal computer
programmable arrays from architectural software
computed to endpoint outcome.

It is difficult to see the physical brain and its nerves without preconceptions. Yet, if we are to move forward, we must close our eyes, and open them back up as if we are seeing the nervous system for the very first time. To see the physical brain without those rules that lock us in is to see something NEW. Therefore, to observe that the nerve system is the system through which the innate law centralizes and transmits innate impulses for coordination of action in animal bodies is to delve into the area WHERE there can be interference with TRANSMISSION of information/F (pri. 12, 29).

In order to explain this old observation in a NEW way, parallel logic will be utilized to facilitate the understanding of our induction. To emphasize again, the maxim, *"we cannot give what we do not own"* is true. Whatever we "construct" into EXTERNAL structural forms is ALWAYS a reflection of INTERNAL living systems. This explains clearly why we can use any external educated constructs to rely on them as being a reflection any innate internal innate constructs. This is the reason why when we observe computer data processing systems, what we observe are external educated constructs that truly reflect internal innate constructs. For example, living, thinking E/matter already exists in the universe and is alive in us (pri. 1, 20, 23). It is a component of WHO we are as human beings. That is WHY we can actualize the many EXTERNAL structural forms that we live with in the world. Examples abound, we invented the water pump (heart), bridges (ligaments), filter (nose), artificial breathing machine (lungs), camera (eye), telephone (ear), irrigation (circulatory system), data processing systems (brain and nerves), etc... Metabolism of tissue cells, coordination of activities of body parts, and voluntary actions is demonstrated in the next flowchart *(see diagram 3).*

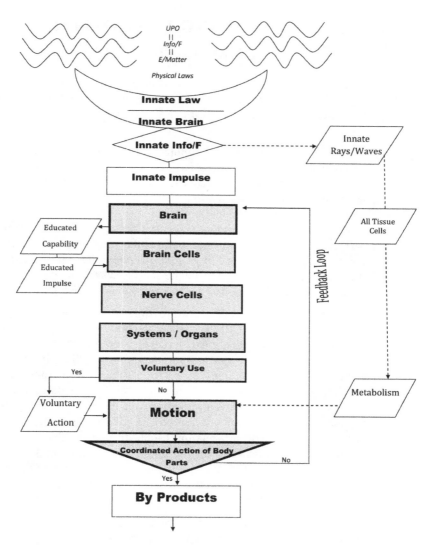

Diagram 3:
Flowchart of the innate law of vertebrate adapting
information/F and E/matter for use in the body through
metabolism using innate rays; for coordination of action using innate
impulses; for voluntary actions using educated impulses
(tinctured innate impulses).

FOLLOWING THE NORMAL
COMPLETE CYCLE

The universal principle of organization and the innate law of living things are the starting points of our observation regarding the human body (Step 1 and 2 of the "Normal Complete Cycle" for coordination of activities).

The body is akin to a SUPER computer. It requires an operating system to be used by the innate law. The innate law is 100%/perfect normal software (pri. 22, 27) that is CONTINUALLY, moment by moment, computing, coding, and adapting, information/F and E/matter for use in the body and coordinating the activities of all the parts of the body (pri. 23). Stephenson wrote, "This force or message is specific for the momentary needs of a tissue cell".[1: p.265] As mentioned before, the operating system is called the innate field (brain) and it is non-discrete. The innate field, which is the operating system of the innate law, is where innate impulses are assembled, and that it is located wherever the innate law is.

By definition ALL processes require time (pri. 6), and consequently coordination of action of all the parts of the body (pri. 23, 32) is a process that requires time. Coordination of action also requires the INSTRUCTIVE information/F from the innate law, which is a 100% instructive act (100%/Perfect Innate Realm," step 3) to be conducted from a physical centralizing center, which is the physical brain, to the parts of the body at the periphery. It needs centralization and distribution from center to periphery. Time is paramount for physical living E/matter to process instructive data (innate information/F) and to express that "data (pri. 6, 13 and 21). It requires time for the innate law, as normal 100%/perfect innate software (pri. 22, 27), using the material hardware of the body, to compute instructive information/F (pri. 23) that **is possible** in accordance with universal laws (pri. 24).

It is enough to say that the organizing principle, through the expression of its instructive data by physical E/matter (pri. 13) and its manifested physical motion (pri. 14), must interface with each other. This interface is the union of the non-discrete principle and physical E/matter expressing instructive information/F **organized** by the universal principle of organization (pri. 10). The next step is for the innate law to compute, code, and adapt information/F (pri. 23) through its operating system, called the innate field; then innate information/F is centralized within the physical brain ("Brain Cell", step 4) for coordination of activities. From the innate field as control center, the innate law characterizes those innate impulses through network interface ("Innate Characterization", step 5) and then TRANSMITS them through neurological E/matter (transmitters) to ALL the parts of the body for coordination of action (pri. 23).

It requires time to compute data ("Transformation/Coding," step 6), for the data to be processed by living E/matter (pri. 6). Computation between different parts must be interconnected with each other through a network of nerves. These innate impulses (data) are centralized within a specific central processing unit (CPU) to provide coherence of their specific instructions for coordinated activity. A CPU is the programmed circuitry within a computer that carries out the instruction of a computer software program. In the body this programmed circuitry is the physical brain and the software program is the 100%/perfect innate law. Thus, it is the innate law of living things that is the software and it is 100%/perfect (pri. 5, 7, 22,) and normal (pri. 27). This innate law software is specifically computing, coding, and adapting universal information/F into innate impulses by performing the basic, logical control of input/output (I/O) operations that are specified by its instructions. The central processing unit (CPU) within any vertebrate animal body is the physical brain comprised of conductive E/matter. It consists of a specialized system of nerve cells, basically micro-controllers and micro-processors, that are comprised of specialized neurons. These neurons can transmit information/F in the form of an innate impulse through a conductor ("Innate Impulse," step 7). This specialized system is necessary to first centralize, in the physical brain (CPU), the already assembled innate impulses from the innate field (OS) and then to propel them ("Propulsion," step 8) to the different parts of the body.

Of the many tissues in the vertebrate animal body, the central nervous system, with its brain, spinal cord and nerves, comprise the interconnective wiring network, which the innate law adapts to communicate its coded instructions to all of the different parts of the body for coordination of activities (pri. 28). These coded instructions from the innate law become coordinates of kinematics motions. This, in turn, facilitates the transmission of innate impulses in compliance with the principle of coordination (pri. 32). From the adaptation of the E/matter of the central nervous system by the innate law (pri. 23), innate information/F is in-forming neurons into specific applications. These neurons are constructed into a multitude of data processing circuits (microprocessors) interfacing with each other. Remember that external educated constructs are simply a reflection of internal innate constructs. It is the innate law (100%/perfect innate software) that governs the interface computation through the innate field (OS) to centralize the already assembled innate impulses within the physical brain (CPU).

From the physical brain (CPU), the innate law adapts and controls a network of nerves as transmitter hardware agents ("Efferent Nerve," step 9) to distribute the data by transmitting the innate impulses ("Transmission," step 10), which are the instructions, through conductive E/matter to the all parts of the body at the periphery ("Tissue Cell," step 11 and "Reception," step 12). These parts in turn are adapted with specific analytical non-discrete device drivers that are peripheral integrated circuits governed by the innate law to decode the instructions of the innate impulses at the periphery, for the coordination of actions of the parts of the body (pri. 23, 32). Those device drivers are within the innate field, which is EVERYWHERE the innate law is located, and they are non-discrete.

Stephenson calls this decoding activity, "Physical Personification" since he ascribed the pronoun "she" to the innate law. It is actually the manifesting motion (pri. 14) ("Physical Representation," step 13). This representation is an interface of the non-physical and physical and it occurs through the function of information/F that is to **unite** the organizing law with E/matter (pri. 10). All this is so extremely complex that the interface itself is separate and distinct (pri. 4). The interface is a part OF and a part FROM the innate law of living things, information/F and E/matter.

The innate law acts through a highly specialized computer system (i.e., body of a living thing) using an intricate network of communication for the purpose of coordination of action of all the parts of the body (pri. 23, 32). The central nervous system is the transmitting inter-connective network through which the innate law coordinates the action of all the interoperable parts of the body for mutual benefit ("Expression," step 14). Those parts also INCLUDE the cells of the central nervous system. It must be remembered that the central nervous system also needs coordinated action. The central nervous system is comprised of living E/matter, called neurons, continually adapted by the innate law to perform specific functions along with all of the other tissue cells ("Function," step 15). Coordination of activities requires a feedback mechanism that will inform the physical brain (CPU) of the response of the receptor body part for coordination of activities. There is coordination within the receptor body part that will ultimately give rise to coordination of ALL the parts of the living body through interoperability ("Coordination", steps 16). The coordination of activities of the receptor cells of the body part will in turn manifest motion ("Tissue Cell," step 17). There are many similarities between computer processing and body processing. Of course the body is controlled by a 100%/perfect innate software and expresses signs of life; it is self-organizing, self-adapting and self-healing. A computer does not have that ability. The body is a super computer that is comprised of analytical device drivers within the innate filed, which are operated and controlled by the innate law. These device drivers are non-discrete and are controlled by the innate law in order to recode feedback information/F from the receptor body part. This feedback information/F is from the motion brought about by the action of the receptor body part and to be transmitted back to the central processing unit, the physical brain ("Vibration," step 18). At this precise moment, the NEW coded impulse that is assembled within the innate field, which is EVERYWHERE the innate law is located, provides specific instructions to non-discrete markers and device drivers that will program the conducting E/matter ("Impression/Recoding", step 19). This computation will adapt the neurons for proper transmission back to the physical brain-CPU ("Trophic Impluse", step 20). The conducting E/matter is carrying the coded-feedback from the receptor body part ("Afferent Nerves," step 21), which is a specific impression of vibration to transmit the feedback ("Transmission," step 22) to the physical brain ("Brain Cell," step 23).

Once the physical brain receives this NEW coded feedback from the body part ("Reception," step 24), the innate law will then decode and transform this information/F through perfect innate processing ("100%/Perfect Innate Realm," step 25) to interpret its message ("Interpretation," step 26). At this level, a series of integrated physical circuits, in the form of brain cells grouping within the physical brain (CPU), will sense the feedback of the body part ("Sensation/Feedback," step 27). This feedback will be decoded into information/F from the innate law, and received by the physical brain (CPU), ("Integral Innate Processing," step 28). All conducted information/F is CONTINUALLY computed by the innate law ("Innate Law of Living Things," step 29) for the purpose of coordination of action of all the parts for mutual benefit (pri. 23). It is then that the innate law constructs NEW coded impulses relating to the specific parameters of the body parts for coordination of activities if it is possible according to universal laws ("100%/Perfect Instantaneous Integral Adaptation," step 30). The adaptation that universal information/F and E/matter relating to the parameters of the body part brings us back to the fundamental organizing principle ("Universal Principle of Organization," step 31), finalizing the NORMAL COMPLETE CYCLE for coordination of activities.

It must be noted that steps 16 through 31 are the same steps in reverse, using similar components with the afferent nerves as a feedback loop of the innate law to CONTINUALLY adapt information/F and E/matter specific to the parameters of the body part moment to moment for coordination of actions (pri. 23, 32).

Note to the student: Innate information/F can be *conducted* to govern coordination of action or can be *radiated* to govern the cellular components for metabolism. Chiropractic addresses **ONLY** the transmission of **CONDUCTED** innate information/F for coordination of activities.

Re-contextualized, principle #28 states:

No. 28. THE CONDUCTORS OF INNATE INFORMATION/F.

THE CONDUCTED INFORMATION/F OF THE INNATE LAW OF LIVING THINGS OPERATES THROUGH OR OVER THE NERVOUS SYSTEM IN ANIMAL BODIES.

29

No. 29. Interference with Transmission of Innate Forces. There can be interference with the transmission of Innate forces.

In the 1920s Stephenson wrote, "We have seen that universal forces can suffer interference with transmission (pri. 12) whether they are radiant or conducted. Innate forces are no exception to the rule and so there can be interference with their transmission through or over the nervous system".[1: p.295] Let us remember that the nervous system is a transmitter of conducted innate impluse that is used ONLY for coordination of action of all the parts of the body. Stephenson also wrote, "If a nerve is made abnormal in any part (as by impingement) there cannot be normal function of that nerve cell, which is a living organism. The mental impulse is robbed of some of its values... it no longer is a perfectly considerate Innate force". [1: p.295-298] When the innate impulse loses its momentum of transmission, its instructive data (message) becomes corrupted and it is no longer an innate information/F for constructive purposes.

With the knowledge of the 2020s, we understand that the innate impulse is a computed, coded, and adapted information/F. It is established that force, in chiropractic, is information/F. It is consistent with Stephenson when he wrote, "The mental impulse is not an energy at all. It is a message. A message is not a material, an energy, or a thing physical in any sense".[1: p.294] When a nerve cell is impinged, it is NOT at ease; it will not transmit the innate impulse properly. There will be a change in momentum of the transmission due to an improper function of the nerve cell that will cause a change in the character of the innate impulse. The receptor part of the body will then receive a modified message that carries misinformation due to its improper timing (pri. 6). This in turn will alter coordination of action. Therefore, the impingement causes the conducting E/matter (nerve cell-transmitter) to react and to lose its ability to transmit the innate impulse in a timely manner. The result is an interference with the transmission of conducted innate information/F. The transmission of coded data (information/F) can be interfered with through transmitters. "Interference may prevent reception altogether, may cause only a temporary loss of signal, or may affect the quality of the sound or picture produced by your equipment. The two most common causes of interference are transmitters and electrical equipment".[19] For an example of signal interference, *(See diagram 4).*

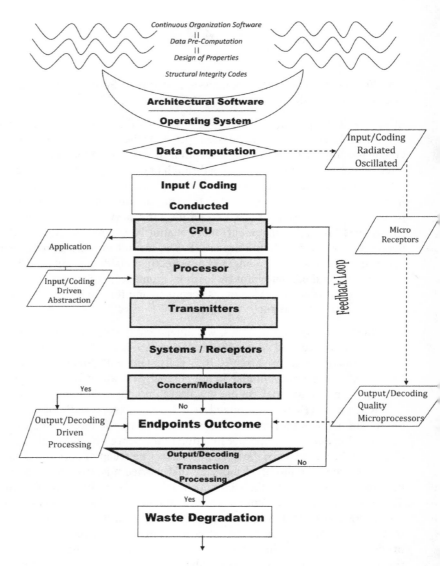

Diagram 4:
Flowchart of the universal computer programmable
arrays from architectural software computed to endpoint
outcome with interference of transmitters.

The code of the innate impulse is reverted back to its original universal state due to the altered momentum in transmission. It returns to being an unadapted universal information/F that is deconstructive toward structural E/matter (pri. 26) and causes an imbalance of information/F in the body. Stephenson wrote, "It has proportion of quality which is nothing less than mere unadapted universal forces, unable to balance properly the universal forces, *ALREADY* in the Tissue Cell (emphasis mine) (pri. 1, 14)".[1: p.296] Should these forces be withdrawn, "the living organisms revert back to the elemental state wherein their molecules act according to the unswerving laws of physics and chemistry."[1: p.268]

Within the chiropractic science context, studies have shown that, "A pressure of only 10mm Hg produced a significant conduction block, the potential falling to 60% of its initial value in 15 minutes and to half its initial value in 30 minutes."[26] When the interference with transmission of the conducting nerve cell occurs, it lacks ease and becomes imbalanced due to its impingement. Then the nerve cell cannot convey the innate impulse with normal momentum and a pivotal moment happens at the site of the impingement. This altered momentum reverts the adapted innate information/F (innate impulse) that is constructive toward structural E/matter to an unadapted universal information/F (nerve impulse) that is deconstructive toward structural E/matter (pri. 26). The lack of ease corrupts the data of the nerve cell altering the momentum of transmission. Stephenson wrote it this way, "A nerve cell which is impinged is not a cell 'at ease.' Therefore, it will not 'vibrate' normally in function. Its function is to convey the message. If it does not function properly it does not carry the 'urge' *(momentum)* properly, therefore the tissue receives a message, which does not 'read true'."[1: p.299-300]

Note to the student: The parts (organs, glands, vessels, etc...) of the body are not dumb or smart; they simply are biophysical agents expressing the information/F that they receive. Junk in, junk out, so to speak.

Re-contextualized, principle #29 states:

No. 29. INTERFERENCE WITH TRANSMISSION OF CONDUCTED INNATE INFORMATION/F.

THERE CAN BE INTERFERENCE WITH THE TRANSMISSION OF CONDUCTED INNATE INFORMATION/F.

30

No. 30. The Causes of Dis-ease. Interference with the transmission of Innate forces causes incoordination of dis-ease.

In the 1920s Stephenson wrote, *"Dis-ease* is a Chiropractic term meaning not having ease; or lack of ease. It is lack of entity. It is a condition of matter when it does not have the property of ease. Ease is the entity, and *dis-ease* the lack of it".[1: p.302]

With the knowledge of the 2020s, observation shows that a transmitting nerve cell that is impinged by a vertebral subluxation for a period of time will be deprived of its ease as regard to its function.[1: p.299-300] It will be in a state of **DIS-EASE**. It is lacking ease.[1: p.302] The nerve cell, as a transmitter, has failed to decode the necessary instructive message of its own innate impulse and to transmit it properly. A nerve cell (transmitter) in a state of **DIS-EASE** due to impingement will not properly transmit innate impulses from brain cell (CPU) to the receiving cells of the part (receptor). It must be STRONGLY emphasized that this interference in transmission is between CPU-brain cell and receiving tissue cell of the body part (receptor). The interference in transmission is between E/matter and E/matter and NOT between the innate principle and E/matter. "Why?" the student may ask? Because if the interference was between the organizing principle and E/matter, E/matter would cease to be **maintained** in existence! This is not possible according to the principles of chiropractic's basic science (pri. 1, 2, 3, 4, 5, 24). Chiropractic is ALWAYS about what is possible EXCLUSIVELY. The student must keep in mind that the innate law of living things is simply the essential extension of the universal principle of organization that has become specifically adaptive for the body of living things. The innate law of living things gives rise to a different organizational state of E/matter. It is within the transmitter-nerve cell that the interference occurs. The function of the conducting E/matter is now interfered with. The lack of ease of a transmitter-nerve cell alters the momentum of the transmission of innate impulses that violates the principle of coordination (pri. 32). The result of this interference is in-coordination of **DIS-EASE**. Further along the path of the innate impulse, the receiving body part (receptor) will then lack coordination of action. Thus, the lack of ease of the transmitter-nerve cell leads to in-coordination, hence the term, "in-coordination of dis-ease".[1: p.xxxiii]

Within the chiropractic science context, chiropractors recognize that "flow" of innate information/F through the nerve cell, "in both directions at the same time, include information molecules".[27: p.255-272] Therefore, when the impingement on the transmitter-nerve cell occurs at the vertebral level, the momentum of the "flow" of innate impulse is disrupted due to the lack of ease of the transmitter-nerve cell that is reverting the innate impulse back "to its elemental state". Innate information/F reverts back to an unadapted universal information/F and is deconstructive toward structural E/matter (pri. 26).

Re-contextualized, principle #30 states:

No. 30. THE CAUSES OF DIS-EASE.

INTERFERENCE WITH TRANSMISSION OF CONDUCTED INNATE INFORMATION/F CAUSES INCOORDINATION OF DIS-EASE.

31

No. 31. Subluxations. Interference with transmission in the body is always directly or indirectly due to subluxations in the spinal column.

In the 1920s Stephenson wrote, "Chiropractic is a science of the cause – not effects".[1: p.93] He also wrote, "A subluxation impinging a nerve from brain to organ, also impinges the nerve supplying its own tissues; that is why it exists as a subluxation."[1: p.309] Dr. Stephenson wrote the definition of vertebral subluxation in his text of 1927, and it is a complete definition. It is clear. It is unadulterated. It is the major focus of attention of the chiropractic objective. Stephenson was clear, "A subluxation is a condition of a vertebra that has lost its proper juxtaposition with the one above, or the one below, or both; to an extent less than a luxation; and which impinges nerves and interferes with the transmission of mental impulses. All the factors of the foregoing definition must be included in order that it be a Chiropractic definition."[1: p.320] Therefore, it is when all the vertebra are in *right relationship* that the momentum of flow of innate impulses is INNATE NORMAL (pri. 27), meaning that it is WITHOUT any interference in transmission (pri. 29), thus it satisfies the principle of coordination (pri. 32).

With the knowledge of the 2020s, if the third law of motion stating that every action has an opposite and equal reaction is applied, it can be seen that the encoded instructive data (message) of the innate impulse maintains the structural integrity of the all the vertebra of the spine in proper balance. If the internal resistance of the body, due to limitation of E/matter, is overcome by an external invasive universal information/F, there will be an imbalance causing a vertebral subluxation. "A subluxation is an abnormality produced in the body by resistive force in response to an external force. It is not produced by the direct application of the external force. A force which results in the subluxation of a vertebra very seldom strikes it."[1: p.322] When the resistance is overcome, the reaction to the internal resistance is unbalanced and the muscles from WITHIN the body will then derange the vertebra thus causing a vertebral subluxation. The subluxated vertebra will impinge the transmitter-nerve cell producing a lack of ease. It is the lack of ease of the transmitter-nerve cell that is called DIS-EASE and is CAUSED by a vertebral subluxation.

Within the chiropractic science context, a nerve cell that does not conduct innate impulses properly will lose its ability to convey the encoded information/F to the receiving body part (receptor) through synaptic transmission and ephaptic response. "Ephatic responses are observed following blockage of action potential... that can elicit excitation in nerves creating a reverberating cycle affecting muscle tone."[28: p26] Even though chiropractic NEVER addresses trauma, it must ne noted that according to Stephenson, "Nerves can be impinged by abnormal positions of bodily parts, by broken bones, by prolapsed organs, by tumors, and by scar tissue. But unless these causes are of traumatic origin, the primary cause is traceable to the spinal foramina or spinal canal, where misplaced vertebrae are impinging fibers."[1: p.308] An indirect pressure of a nerve cell coming from prolapsed organs, tumors, and scar tissue is, in and of itself, CAUSED by vertebral subluxations, unless these abnormal events are due to trauma. Chiropractic does not address trauma. It is for this reason that the interference in transmission of conducted innate information/F in the body is always *directly* or *indirectly* due to a vertebral subluxation; the interference in transmission is the CAUSE of DIS-EASE within the transmitter-nerve cell. The transmitter-nerve cell is now lacking ease.

It is known that innate information/F operates through or over the nerve system in animal bodies (pri. 28). It is understood that the interference with TRANSMISSION of conducted innate information/F takes place within the transmitter-nerve cell, between the CPU-brain cell and the intended receiving body part (receptor). It must be STRONGLY emphasized, once again, that this interference in transmission is between brain cell and tissue cell of the body part, in other words, between E/matter and E/matter, NOT between the innate principle and E/matter. The reason is that if the interference were between the innate principle and E/matter, E/matter would cease to be **maintained** in existence! And this of course is NOT possible according to the principles of chiropractic's basic science. Chiropractic is always about what is possible.

Vertebrate bodies possess a spinal column, which is comprised of several juxtaposed articulating vertebra to protect the spinal cord, which is the major link, along with its adjacent nerves, between the brain and the parts of the body for their coordination of action for mutual benefit (pri. 23). The vertebra are made of hard bones forming the spinal column protecting this major link of data communication in order to satisfy the principle of coordination of action (pri. 32). These hard bony vertebrae interrelate through a series of articulations. There is an "innate normal" **relationship** of these articulations (pri. 27). It is when these articulations DO NOT properly interrelate and impinge the nerve cell that the interference with TRANSMISSION of innate impulses may occur within the transmitter-nerve cell. It is called a vertebral subluxation.

It must be noted that the interference of innate information/F happens WITHIN the transmitting E/matter between brain cell and the cells of the body part. It is the lack of proper articulations of the hard bony vertebrae of the spinal column that impinges the nerve and changes the **momentum** flow of the innate impulse. This is a vertebral subluxation and it alters the transmitter-nerve cell of the nervous system resulting in an interference of the TRANSMISSION of the innate impulse (pri. 29). The CHANGE of the configuration and velocity of electrons, protons, and neutrons of the TRANSMITTING physical E/matter (nerve cell) prevents EASE of TRANSMISSION of innate impulses, thus corrupting the data due to a change in **momentum.**

At this precise moment, the transmitter-nerve cell is in a state of DIS-EASE and interferes with the TRANSMISSION of conducted innate information/F, which is computed and encoded innate impulses carrying an instructive message. The lack of EASE of the TRANSMITTING physical E/matter (nerve cell) changes the momentum of the transmission which reverts the innate impulse, which is an innate information/F that is constructive as regards to structural E/matter (pri. 26), to a nerve impulse that is an un-adapted universal information/F that is deconstructive as regards to structural E/matter (pri. 26).[1: p.296] When any part of the body receives a nerve impulse instead of an innate impulse, that part will have incoordination of action due to the deconstructive nature of the un-adapted nerve impulse (pri. 26). It is for this reason that principle #30 reads: "incoordination **OF** DIS-EASE" (emphasis mine).[1: p.xxxiii]

It is the impingement of the transmitter-nerve cell that CAUSES a lack of EASE and interferes with the TRANSMISSION of the innate impulse. The transmitter-nerve cell is NOT conveying the instructive message with ease any longer because the momentum is altered due to its lack of ease. The transmitter-nerve cell is in a state of DIS-EASE due to the vertebral subluxation; this, in turn, increases the limitations of E/matter of the body. The lack of ease of the transmitter-nerve cell causes E/matter to be more limited than before the subluxation, and it CAUSES in-coordination of action of any receiving parts of the body (pri. 23, 24). Thus, this interference with transmission of innate information/F causes incoordination **of** DIS-EASE (pri. 30).

Re-contextualized, principle #31 states:

No. 31. VERTEBRAL SUBLUXATIONS.

INTERFERENCE WITH TRANSMISSION OF CONDUCTED INNATE INFORMATION/F IS ALWAYS DIRECTLY OR INDIRECTLY DUE TO VERTEBRAL SUBLUXATIONS.

32

No. 32. The Principle of Coordination. Coordination is the principle of harmonious action of all the parts of an organism, in fulfilling their offices and purposes.

In the 1920s, Stephenson had once again a new insight and wrote, "Then, Innate Intelligence is the coordinating principle".[1: p.322] On the previous page he had written, "It is not fully understood what mental impulses are." Regardless of not fully understanding what innate impulses are, the fact remains that the innate law of living things coordinates that which is not understood by us at the moment. This is because the innate law of living things is 100%/perfect (pri. 22) for ALL living E/matter.

With the knowledge of the 2020s, it is now known that the innate impulse is encoded information/F by the innate law through adaptive computation, and provides instructions for coordination of actions (pri. .23, 32). According to Hans Selye, 1946, and more recently Paul H. Black, 1994, that general adaptation occurs through neurotransmitters that exist for bidirectional interactions between the CNS and the immune system.[29: p.1-6] The coordination of ALL activities of ALL the systems of the body is governed by the innate law, the function of which is, to adapt information/F and E/matter that can be used by the body (pri. 23).

Within the chiropractic science context, innate computation of universal information/F is an adaptation encoding an infinite number of innate impulses as *input* instructions for coordination of action of ALL the parts of the body as *output*. For example, "Picking up a glass of beer in a bar does not seem a difficult task. Yet, the apparent ease with which we execute this action obscures the complex tasks our motor system has to solve when organizing this drinking action. In fact, the motor system has to organize the action at different levels. For the realization of movement to the glass, the reach has to be coordinated with the grasping component to bring the hand in the proper configuration to the right place. When one lifts the glass, the load and grip forces applied by the fingers have to be coordinated to account for the weight of the glass, its fragility, and possible slippage, etc, etc..."[30: p.70] This example uses voluntary functions. "It is used by Innate, by virtue of experience and training stored within it, as an organ to so 'tincture' impulses that they are *consciously* guided --- called voluntary functions".[1: p162] It is the innate law that encodes ALL of the innate impulses, as a proprioception *input,* providing innate information/F in the form of instructions to the educated brain about the current position of the limb in relation to the predictions based on the internal representation for *output.* It is an educated function requiring voluntary actions. In fact, the tinctured educated impulse is propelled from the CPU-brain cell to the transmitter-nerve cell in order to convey the tinctured innate instructive information/F, which is an educated impulse for voluntary actions. Coordination of activities relies on multiples agents interacting toward a common objective, that of coherent actions of all the information/F processing systems of the body (pri. 23, 24). "In systems neuroscience, synchronized subthreshold and suprathreshold oscillatory neuronal activity within and between neuronal assemblies is acknowledged as a fundamental mode of neuronal information processing".[31: p.8] It is indeed about coherence, meaning a consistent balance of actions. Otherwise, as Stephenson wrote, "When the pseudo mental impulse arrives at the tissue cell, it is not the perfectly assembled unit that Innate started out on the journey to the cell. It has a proportion of quality which is nothing less than mere unadapted universal forces, unable to *balance* (emphasis mine) properly the universal forces, already in the Tissue Cell (pri. 1, 14)".[1: p.202,296] Coherent synchronization requires feedback for coordination of activities. A fundamental element of coordination of action is to have a feedback loop, which is the Normal Complete Cycle.[1: p.11]

Coordination tasks result from the computations of the innate law governing the momentum of the FLOW of transmission of innate impulses necessary for coherent activities of all the parts of the body (pri. 23, 32) *(See diagram 4).*

Re-contextualized, principle #32 states:

No. 32. THE PRINCIPLE OF COORDINATION.

COORDINATION IS THE PRINCIPLE OF COHERENT ACTIONS OF ALL THE PARTS OF AN ORGANISM IN FULFILLING THEIR ROLES AND PURPOSES.

33

No. 33. The Law of Demand and Supply. The Law of Demand and Supply is existent in the body in its ideal state; wherein the "clearing house," is the brain, Innate the virtuous "banker," brain cells "clerks," and nerve cells "messengers.

In the 1920s Stephenson wrote, "In order that Innate may make demand of all the tissue cells under her jurisdiction, in harmony with organization, she must receive the demands from all the tissue cells in order to know their needs".[1: p.334] The reason Stephenson reasoned this way came from the anthropomorphic personification of innate intelligence. According to him, "she" thinks like you and me, "she" needs to know what going on to make demands, and "she" lived in the physical brain, like a goddess, to control all the needs of the cells.

Throughout his textbook, Dr. Stephenson did not differentiate between different levels of organization. He did not relate to the innate law of the cell, the innate law of the organ, the innate law of the system, the innate law of the body. According to Stephenson, every need of the cell was supplied by the "mental" impulse.[1: p.59] Yet, he did acknowledged, that the "mental force may be radiated".[1: p.31] from within each cell. Now, because of organ transportation for transplants, we know about the innate law of the organ. This innate information/F is called a mental ray. A mental ray is an adapted universal information /F for use in the body; it is responsible to control the cellular components for the metabolism of the cell, of the organ, of the system and of the body to be maintained **as living**. Obviously, coordination of action of anything is NOT necessary for the body to be maintained alive. After all, some of ourbody parts may be absent or may be expressing incoordination of action at this very moment and we are still alive.

What is the parameter of the cell to be maintained as living? It is metabolism of the cell that is effectuated by mental rays that are computed, encoded, and assembled, within the innate field (OS) by the innate law (100%/ perfect normal software), which is located EVERYWHERE in the body. These mental rays are then radiated from within each individual cell from the innate law of the cell to control its components from within the cell itself. The same applies to all the different levels of organization of living E/matter (i.e., cells, organs, systems, and bodies).

With the knowledge of the 2020s, it is understood that there is a perfect innate processing within the body of a living thing to adapt to any internal or external environmental circumstances if it is possible according to universal laws (pri. 24). This means that the innate law acts precisely as a 100%/perfect NORMAL software (pri. 22, 27), that is ALWAYS updated moment to moment. It is continually governing EVERY single process of the body. The innate law has no specific location within the body; it is EVERYWHERE about the body. This is because there is 100%/perfect organization at the cell level, organ level, system level and body level. The law of demand and supply was a good analogy for Stephenson's understanding in his time using anthropomorphism. Today, there is the obligation to update the analogy according to the NEW knowledge available in the 21st Century.

The universal principle of organization organizes E/matter CONTINUALLY SUPPLYING to it properties and actions, thus **maintaining** it in existence (pri. 1). **It is the starting point of chiropractic's basic SCIENCE. It is the initial and fundamental principle.** CONTINUALLY SUPPLYING is emphasized because the supply of universal information/F is continuous and NEVER missing, otherwise E/matter would cease to be **maintained** in existence. Stephenson wrote, "While Innate is limited as to the amount of matter it controls, which is the amount of matter in the body, she is not limited as to the amount of forces at her command (pri. 9). She has the whole universe to draw from.... When Innate leaves the body, the matter in it is not destroyed but reverts to its inorganic state.... Universal Intelligence is still 'interested' in the molecules, though not in the structures, and still gives these molecules and atoms as much care as ever. If it did not they would cease to exist at all" (pri. 1, 14).[1: p.19] Therefore, the universal principle of organization (pri. 1) is the CAUSE of the laws of conservation of energy, of matter, of information, and other universal laws; it is the universal principle of organization that **maintains** E/matter in existence through the bond of information/F (pri. 10). The universal principle of organization is a fundamental principle that explains other laws and makes them **possible.**

The law of continuous supply and computation is what best describes the NEW analogy of the 2020s. How can any "thing" comprised of atoms, molecules, and cells need to demand whatever when it is **CONTINUALLY** supplied everything in terms of properties and actions in order to be **maintained** in existence? The universal law of gravity does not need demands from atoms and molecules. This universal law **continually** supplies the atoms and molecules with its information/F providing them concrete geometry and attracting them toward the center of the earth. It is the same with the universal laws of motion and conservation. It is the universal principle of organization that **continually** supplies properties and actions to E/matter **maintaining** it in existence (pri. 1), and this fundamental principle is **NOT** dependent on demand. In order to be **maintained** alive, living E/matter must comply within specific levels and parameters of organization of properties and actions. It is the universal principle of organization that **continually** supplies them to **maintain** it in existence and it is its essential extension, the innate law that adapts them to maintain living E/matter alive (pri. 23) within limitations (pri. 24). The innate law of living things is 100%/perfect (pri. 22); it is also normal and its function is also normal (pri. 27). It adapts universal information/F and E/matter for use in the body for mutual benefits of its parts (pri. 23) in accordance with universal laws (pri. 24). Chiropractic ALWAYS deals with CAUSE and NEVER deals with EFFECT. "Chiropractic is a science of cause – not effects.[1: p.93] Therefore, its principles should be directed at CAUSE. The starting point of chiropractic's basic science, principle #1, is what makes **possible** (CAUSE) the subsequent 32 principles as it **maintains** the entire universe in existence. Principle #33 should also be directed at CAUSE. It is imperative that the principles of chiropractic's basic science be formulated at CAUSE and refined in contemporary terminology according to the knowledge that we have available to us in the 2020s which was not known in the 1920s.

The analogy of the "clearing house", "virtuous banker", "clerks" and "messengers" was a very good in 1927. Stephenson's comparison was genius even though it might be hard to find a "virtuous banker" nowadays. The analogy and terminology, however, need to be modernized and re-contextualized. Remember that B.J. used anthropomorphism when referring to innate intelligence as "she." Innate intelligence was the "Big Fellow Upstairs" and educated intelligence was the "Little Fellow Downstairs"[32] Dr. Stephenson even wrote, "This afferent side of the Nine Functions is called by Dr. Palmer, 'The Wife'."[1: p.189-190] It is also well documented that B.J. used of theomorphism in his Green Books, calling universal intelligence "God" and innate intelligence "God in man". Despite being confusing, it is quite understandable why Stephenson selected the Law of Demand and Supply, used in human socio-economic affairs, as an analogy for principle #33 and actually called Innate the "virtuous banker." He simply continued the use of anthropomorphism for the analogy of principle #33. It was NOT wrong during the early developments of chiropractic. It is, however, outdated given the NEW knowledge of the 21st century.

As educated intelligence grows, more knowledge is acquired and understanding develops proportionally. In Stephenson's textbook it reads, "As Chiropractic grows older and people's knowledge of nerve physiology increases, more is known about the afferent nerves, and year by year the findings of the anatomist support the Chiropractic theories along this line"[1: p.55] Marcel Proust (French novelist, critic, essayist, 1871-1922) was one of the most influential writers of the 20th century is quoted, "The real voyage of discovery consists not in seeing new landscape but in having new eyes."[33] Today, we see the OLD (1920s) through the lens of NEW (2020s).

Computer science provides six categories of computational principles, most of which are analogous to chiropractic. According to Peter Denning, computer scientist, they are: "Computation (meaning and limits of computing), Communication (reliable data transmission), Coordination (networked entities toward common goals), Recollection (storage and retrieval of information), Evaluation (performance prediction and capacity planning), Design (building reliable computing systems)"[34: p.16] *(See diagram 5)*

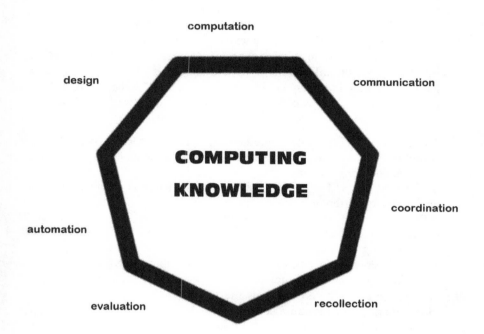

[Excerpt] Figure 1. Categories of the Great Principles (GP) framework

Diagram 5:
Computation categories of computing knowledge space into
windows to see structures and behavior of field elements

Computation, communication, coordination, recollection, automation, evaluation, and design can be used as an updated analogy for principle #33. Computation is UNIVERSAL. According to Michael Levet from the University of South Carolina, Dept of Mathematics, "It is also important to note that there are numerous models of computation that are vastly different none are more powerful than the UNIVERSAL Turing machine. The Turing machine is the only machine that needs to be studied."[35: p.93-95] Automation is "the state of being operated automatically." Communication is "exchange of information". Coordination is "the coherent and harmonious functioning of parts for effective results." Recollection is "the action of recalling of processes." Evaluation is "to determine." Design is "to have a purpose."

The Universality Principle of the Universal Turing Machine is used with computers stating that, "A general computer is capable of performing any computation that any other computer can."[36: p.95] The importance of the UNIVERSAL Turing Machine is clear. There is no need to have an infinity of different machines doing different jobs. A single one will suffice. According to Alan Turing himself, "The engineering problem of producing various machines for various jobs is replaced by the office work of 'programming' the UNIVERSAL machine to do these jobs."[37: p.4] This is, of course, only possible because of computing, which according to Oxford Dictionary, "is not physically existing as such but made by software to appear to do so." This literally means that it takes place in a virtual world, which is non-discrete. This will become clear as we develop our analogy with the computer. The innate law is the only software that needs to be studied, in regards to living things.

Universality holds only in this virtual world. Computers are sometimes said to be universal in the world of computation. If we look at computers as real machines and not only virtual machines, they depend very much on their environments. They require a CONTINUOUS SUPPLY of electricity, they must be handled with care, they must not be exposed to extreme temperature, and so forth. In other words, they have limitations of their own materials.

Philosopher John Searle asked the question: "Can the operation of the brain be simulated on a digital computer?" Then he answered his question this way, "The answer seems to me... demonstrably 'Yes'... That is, naturally interpreted the question means: Is there some description of the brain such that under that description you could do a computational simulation of the operations of the brain. But given the[Turing machine] that anything that can be given a precise enough characterization as a set of steps can be simulated on a digital computer, it follows trivially that the question has an affirmative answer."[38: p.200]

In fact, computing is processing information, whether universal, innate, or educated. Stephenson wrote, "but in the body with an infinite intelligence in charge, it has approached the perfect very closely; the only limitations being that of matter (pri. 24). Application of this principle will show what coordination is and how necessary Intellectual Adaptation and adaptation are. It shows the union and close relation of all these thirty-three principles and any more which we care to derive from them. It binds them together in an unbeatable unit – and that unit is the Essence of Chiropractic."[1: p.333-334] Stephenson is pointing out that the 33 principles are the compass, the GPS (*G*uiding *P*rinciple *S*ystem) if you will, for chiropractors to follow in order to stay on course for practicing "the Essence of Chiropractic." Stephenson says, "The principles of a science are its governing laws."[1: p.xxix] Remember that the innate law of living things is always normal (pri. 27) and always 100%/perfect (pri. 7, 22) and as such it is a law that **continually** governs all operations with in the innate field so it is **continually** 100%/perfect moment by moment in order to compute information/F and E/matter to maintain the body **alive** (pri. 21, 23). The innate law is this 100%/perfect software that never needs updates. It is **continually** up to date, moment to moment, forever and ever!

Look at the Principle of Continuous Supply, which is a principle that continually supplies energy to an in-plant materials supply. According to Robin Hanson, PhD in Technology Management, "With the principle of continuous supply, a number of parts of each part number are presented at the assembly station where they are to be assembled, which means that when continuous supply is used in a mixed-model assembly context, where different assembly objects require different parts, the assembler needs to pick the right part to assemble on each assembly object."[39: p.i]

Stephenson also wrote regarding the innate brain. "That part of the brain used by Innate, as an organ, in which to assemble mental impulses.... Its existence is actual, but its location is theoretical."[1: p.13] The innate field (brain) is non-discrete just like the innate law is non-discrete. The innate field (brain) is located wherever the innate law is located in the body. It is everywhere in the body (cell, organ, system, body, etc...).

As the Law of Continuous Supply and Computation is used for an updated analogy of principle 33, there is now a near perfect analogy that conveys a **continual** supply of information/F within the body. It identifies our universal niche practicing the chiropractic objective, which is to correct subluxations to restore normal transmission of innate impulses.[1: p.270] It also maintains this principle at CAUSE. "Chiropractic is a science of the cause – not effect."[1: p.93]

If Stephenson were around to write his textbook today, he would use a computer for his analogy because our understanding of data processing in the 2020s gives us an opportunity to develop a comparison that is contemporary. It must, however, be kept in mind that although the human body belongs to the Animal Kingdom, humans are much more than animals. Also, although the human body belongs to Category of System Organization, it is much more than computers.

To illustrate further using of the computer analogy. A **C**entral **P**rocessing **U**nit (CPU) is the portion that centralizes control, where all processing ultimately originates from and returns to, even if that unit delegates work to sub-processors. Computers have a CPU for CONTROL purposes, so the computer always knows exactly where or what, in processing terms, it is up to. It is a feedback loop system for coordination of activities.

Based on findings by Sperry & Gazzaniga in 1967, "The brain, unlike the computer does not have a clear CPU. Its neural hierarchy is divided in two hemispheres, each of which receives only half the information and can independently process input and create output, that is, each hemisphere acts like an autonomous brain."[40: p.4] That is why, with the Principle of Continuous Supply and Computation, the operating system (OS) in the analogy is the "innate field" which is non-discrete. The innate field is 100%/perfect and is wherever the innate law is in the body, which is EVERYWHERE.

Let us analyze modern technical communication where the objective is for a computer to transmit a message comprised of coded data through a system. The CPU processes encoded data by software input. The transmitter, through a medium, transmits encoded data from the CPU to a receiver output. The CPU, the transmitter, the medium, and the receiver are physical systems, but the message is not. It is information, initially encoded, assembled, and organized in the computer; then organized and materialized in the CPU; then organized and propelled in the transmitter. What's truly amazing, is that the message can be distinguished with perfect reliability from all other messages as long as there is no interference within the medium of the transmitter. In the words of Alan Turing, "It is my contention that the operations of a computing machine include all those which are used in the computation of a number."[41: p.232]

Within the analogy, the "computer" is the LIVING BODY. The "normal software" (100%/perfect) is the innate law of living thing (pri. 27) that first computes, assembles, encodes, and adapts the information/F (inforuns being information/force units of encoded data) within the "operating system of the computer" which is the INNATE FIELD.[1: p.13] Then comes the interface between discrete and non-discrete (physical and non-physical --- material and non-material) where the innate law computes, encodes, and adapts these inforuns into innate impulses centralizing them in the CPU, which is the PHYSICAL BRAIN. Last, the physical brain-CPU then propels the innate impulse in the transmitters, namely the SPINAL CORD and SPINAL NERVES. This perfect reliability of the message gives rise to the Principle of Coordination for balanced actions and coherence of all the parts of the body (pri. 32).

Note to the student: The innate law also adapts inforuns into innate rays for metabolism of the cell controlling its internal components. Chiropractic does not concern itself with innate rays. Chiropractic is EXLUSIVELY about the restoration of normal transmission of innate impulses for coordination of actions (pri. 23, 32) **(see diagram 3)**.

Re-contextualized, principle #33 states:

No. 33. THE PRINCIPLE OF CONTINUOUS SUPPLY AND COMPUTATION.

THE PRINCIPLE OF CONTINUOUS SUPPLY AND COMPUTATION IS EXISTENT IN THE BODY IN ITS IDEAL STATE; WHEREIN THE LIVING BODY IS THE "COMPUTER," THE INNATE LAW IS THE "NORMAL SOFTWARE," THE INNATE FIELD IS THE "OPERATING SYSTEM," THE PHYSICAL BRAIN IS THE "CENTRAL PROCESSING UNIT," THE BRAIN CELLS ARE THE "PROCESSORS," AND THE NERVE CELLS ARE THE "TRANSMITTERS."

Note to the student: This principle does NOT include the receptor body part receiving the intended message. The receptors are effects. The principles of chiropractic's basic science are at cause.[1: p.93] The 33 principles of chiropractic's basic science are the essence of the body of knowledge of chiropractic.The 33 principles are a description of "WHAT" chiropractic is. The 33 principles of chiropractic's basic science do not speculate on the function of the receptor body part receiving the encoded message. The ONLY concern of chiropractic is that there be NO interference to the transmission of conducted innate information/F that include the message (pri. 29). Chiropractic is about the correction of subluxation for the restoration of the normal flow (momentum) of transmission of innate impulses. IT IS CONTINUALLY ABOVE-DOWN-INSIDE-OUT in the universe. It is a CONTINUOUS ACT through space and time in the universe. It is a universal CONTINUUM forever. It IS the universal principle of organization CONTINUALLY acting ad infinatum and it essential extension, the innate law of living things CONTINUALLY adapting information/F within limitation of E/matter *(See diagram 6)*.

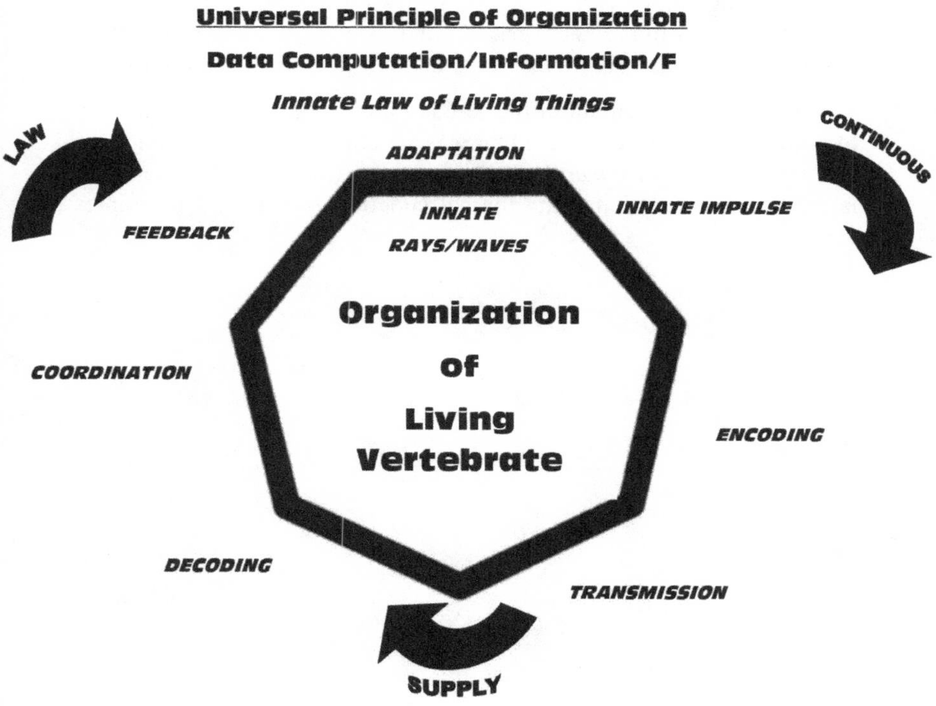

Universal Principle of Organization

Data Computation/Information/F

Innate Law of Living Things

LAW

CONTINUOUS

ADAPTATION

FEEDBACK

INNATE
RAYS/WAVES

INNATE IMPULSE

COORDINATION

**Organization
of
Living
Vertebrate**

ENCODING

DECODING

TRANSMISSION

SUPPLY

Diagram 6:
Computation categories of innate information/F of living
vertebrate for use in the body and coordination of actions
of parts of the body for mutual benefit; these categories
are sustained by the law of *continuous* supply under the
directives of the innate law within the limitation of E/matter.

This analogy can be used to show that the Principle of Continuous Supply and Computation already exists in its ideal state within the living body. It demonstrates the interconnectivity and interoperability of the body parts sharing unlimited possibility of information/F that is included within the principle of continuous supply and computation. In the living body, the principle of continuous supply and computation is governed by the innate law of living things (pri. 20), that is always 100%/perfect and always current, moment to moment (pri. 22), that is always normal (pri. 27), and that is limited by the limitations of E/matter (pri. 24) and time (pri. 6).

This is a NEW refinement of the re-contextualization of the 33 principles of chiropractic's basic science that was demonstrated in 2017 in my book, *A New Look At Chiropractic Basic Science*. It begs the question, "What is the deductive, rational and logical conclusion of the 33 principles of chiropractic's basic science?

THE CHIROPRACTIC OBJECTIVE

If an initial principle is true and we use rational logic with sound deductive reasoning, its subsequent principles and conclusion will also be true! "Chiropractic is a deductive science";[1: p.xvi] therefore, the 33 principles of chiropractic's basic science should reveal the chiropractic objective. The scientific application of the 33 principles, in practice, is actually chiropractic's applied science with its analyses/techniques including the educational programs of practice members. Chiropractic is a complete science.[1: p.xvi] Let us apply some of the principles to see clearly the chiropractic objective:

No. 13. THE FUNCTION OF E/MATTER IS TO EXPRESS INFORMATION/F.

No. 22. THE INNATE LAW OF LIVING THINGS IS ALWAYS 100%/ PERFECT FOR ALL LIVING E/MATTER.

No. 23. THE FUNCTION OF THE INNATE LAW OF LIVING THINGS IS TO ADAPT UNIVERSAL INFORMATION/F AND E/MATTER FOR USE IN THE BODY, SO THAT ALL PARTS OF THE BODY WILL HAVE COORDINATED ACTION FOR MUTUAL BENEFIT.

No. 24. THE INNATE LAW OF LIVING THINGS ADAPTS INFORMATION/F AND E/MATTER FOR THE BODY ONLY IF IT IS POSSIBLE ACCORDING TO UNIVERSAL LAWS.

No. 27. THE INNATE LAW OF LIVING THINGS IS ALWAYS NORMAL AND ITS FUNCTION IS ALWAYS NORMAL.

No. 28. THE CONDUCTED INFORMATION/F OF THE INNATE LAW OF LIVING THINGS OPERATES THROUGH OR OVER THE NERVOUS SYSTEM IN ANIMAL BODIES.

No. 29. THERE CAN BE INTERFERENCE WITH THE TRANSMISSION OF CONDUCTED INNATE INFORMATION/F.

No. 30. INTERFERENCE WITH TRANSMISSION OF CONDUCTED INNATE INFORMATION/F CAUSES INCOORDINATION OF DIS-EASE.

No. 31. INTERFERENCE WITH CONDUCTED INNATE INFORMATION/F IS ALWAYS DIRECTLY OR INDIRECTLY DUE TO VERTEBRAL SUBLUXATIONS.

No. 32. COORDINATION IS THE PRINCIPLE OF COHERENT ACTIONS OF ALL THE PARTS OF AN ORGANISM IN FULFILLING THEIR ROLES AND PURPOSES.

Using deductive reasoning and rational logic, observe that the conclusion of the principles of chiropractic's basic science does reveal the chiropractic objective. Stated: The chiropractic objective is to locate, analyze and facilitate the correction of vertebral subluxations for a normal transmission of the conducted innate information/F of the body. PERIOD. An initial draft of the chiropractic objective first appeared within the objective straight chiropractic lexicon found in the blog called "Chiropractic Outside The Box" (COTB), April 22, 2014.[42] In those days, chiropractors were just beginning to "see" something NEW, to "see" something we never "saw" before. We realized then, that the chiropractic objective stemmed from the view point of E/matter expressing innate information/Forces. Stephenson somewhat identified the chiropractic objective when he wrote, "**The chiropractor aims only to restore** – to bring about restoration."[1: p.270]

The function of E/matter is to express information/F that is governed by the universal principle of organization (pri. 13). Information/F is instruction supplying properties (configurations) and actions (velocities) to the electrons, protons, and neutrons to **maintain** E/matter in existence (pri. 1), uniting the organizing principle with E/matter (pri. 3, 10). As we progress toward more complex levels of organization, we recognize that an essential extension of the universal principle of organization, which is the innate law of living things, is adapting universal information/F and E/matter to maintain the material of the body of a living thing **alive** (pri. 21) within the limitations of E/matter (pri. 24) and of time (pri. 6). The innate law is **ALWAYS** 100%/perfect and complete (pri. 22). The innate law governs living E/matter and is either 100% active or it is 0%; if it has 0% of activity it means that E/matter is dead. There is no in-between with the innate law. It is all (100%) or it is nothing (0%). A thing is alive or it is dead. It is never possible for living E/matter to express more innate law, NEVER! We cannot say that the chiropractic objective is to express more innate. It is the innate law that is the governing principle[1: p.18] and it is **ALWAYS 100%.** The function of E/matter is to express **information/F** (pri. 13) that is organized and governed by the organizing principle (pri. 8). The innate law is non-discrete, meaning immaterial, and is ALWAYS 100%/perfect and complete (pri. 22). Therefore, the correction of vertebral subluxation CANNOT allow E/matter to express more innate. It is NOT possible since the innate law is ALWAYS 100% complete and perfect. The correction of vertebral subluxation allows E/matter to more fully express innate information/F (pri. 13). Remember that the innate law adapts information/F and E/matter for the body **ONLY IF IT IS POSSIBLE** according to universal laws (pri. 24).

However, note the problem. Since the function of E/matter is to express information/F (pri. 13), the expression of information/F by E/matter is an effect and not a cause. Dr. Stephenson wrote, "Chiropractic is a science of cause --- not effects."[1: p.93] Therefore, through rational logic and sound deductive reasoning, for the chiropractic objective to be congruent, it MUST be based on its "science of CAUSE." The chiropractic objective MUST be about bringing restoration.[1: p.270] This begs the question: Restoration of what? And the answer is: The restoration of normal TRANSMISSION of conducted innate information/F through the correction of vertebral subluxations (pri. 27, 28, 29, 31). When the chiropractor has localized, analyzed and facilitated the correction of vertebral subluxations, the work is completed! PERIOD! *(See diagram 7)*.

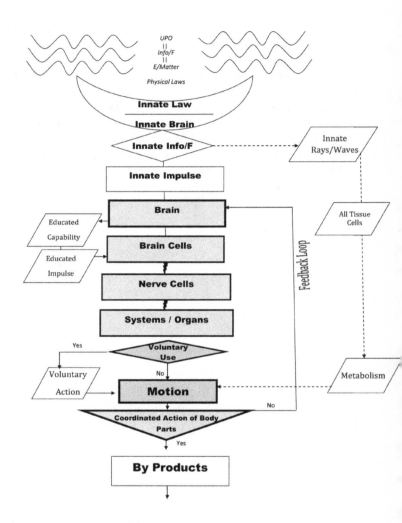

Diagram 7:
Flowchart of the innate law of living vertebrates adapting information/F
and E/matter for use in the body through control of cellular components
for metabolism radiating innate rays/waves within all tissue cells; for
coordination of actions conducting transmission of innate impulses
through the nervous system; for voluntary actions conducting transmission
of educated impulses through the nervous system. It also depicts the
interference with transmission of conducted innate information/F
located within the transmitting nerve cells.The feedback loop is the
necessary communication system EXCLUSIVELY for the control of
coordinated action of all parts of the body for mutual benefit (pri. 23).

Re-contextualized, the chiropractic objective states:

THE CHIROPRACTIC OBJECTIVE.

THE CHIROPRACTIC OBJECTIVE IS TO LOCATE, ANALYZE, AND FACILITATE THE CORRECTION OF VERTEBRAL SUBLUXATIONS FOR A NORMAL TRANSMISSION OF THE CONDUCTED INNATE INFORMATION/F OF THE BODY. PERIOD.

THE 33 PRINCIPLES RE-CONTEXTUALIZED

THIRTY-THREE PRINCIPLES, re-contextualized (2022), numbered and named.

No. 1. THE MAJOR PREMISE.

A UNIVERSAL PRINCIPLE OF ORGANIZATION IS CONTINUALLY SUPPLYING PROPERTIES AND ACTIONS TO ALL E/MATTER, THUS MAINTAINING IT IN EXISTENCE.

No. 2. THE CHIROPRACTIC MEANING OF EXISTENCE.

THE EXPRESSION OF THIS ORGANIZING PRINCIPLE THROUGH E/MATTER IS THE CHIROPRACTIC MEANING OF EXISTENCE.

No. 3. THE UNION OF THE PRINCIPLE OF ORGANIZATION AND E/MATTER.

EXISTENCE IS NECESSARILY THE UNION OF THE UNIVERSAL PRINCIPLE OF ORGANIZATION AND E/MATTER.

No. 4. THE TRIUNE OF EXISTENCE.

EXISTENCE IS A TRIUNITY HAVING THREE NECESSARY UNITED FACTORS, NAMELY, THE PRINCIPLE OF ORGANIZATION, INFORMATION/F AND E/MATTER.

No. 5. THE PERFECTION OF THE TRIUNE.

IN ORDER TO HAVE EXISTENCE, THERE MUST BE 100%/PERFECT ORGANIZING PRINCIPLE, 100%/PERFECT INFORMATION/F AND 100%/PERFECT E/MATTER.

No. 6. THE PRINCIPLE OF TIME.

ALL PROCESSES REQUIRE TIME AND SPACE.

No. 7. THE PERFECTION OF THE ORGANIZING PRINCIPLE IN E/MATTER.

THE PERFECTION OF THE ORGANIZING PRINCIPLE FOR ANY PARTICLE OF E/MATTER IS ALWAYS 100%/PERFECT AND COMPLETE.

No. 8. THE FUNCTION OF THE PRINCIPLE OF ORGANIZATION.

THE FUNCTION OF THE PRINCIPLE OF ORGANIZATION IS TO ORGANIZE INFORMATION/F.

No. 9. THE AMOUNT OF INFORMATION/F.

THE INFORMATION/F ORGANIZED BY THE PRINCIPLE OF ORGANIZATION IS ALWAYS 100%/PERFECT.

No. 10. THE FUNCTION OF INFORMATION/F.

THE FUNCTION OF INFORMATION/F IS TO UNITE THE PRINCIPLE OF ORGANIZATION AND E/MATTER.

No. 11. THE CHARACTER OF UNIVERSAL INFORMATION/F.

THE INFORMATION/F OF THE UNIVERSAL PRINCIPLE OF ORGANIZATION IS MANIFESTED BY PHYSICAL LAWS; IS UNSWERVING AND UNADAPTED, AND HAVE NO SOLICITUDE FOR THE STRUCTURES IN WHICH IT WORKS.

No. 12. INTERFERENCE WITH UNIVERSAL INFORMATION /F.

THERE CAN BE INTERFERENCE WITH THE TRANSMISSION OF UNIVERSAL INFORMATION/F.

No. 13. THE FUNCTION OF E/MATTER.

THE FUNCTION OF E/MATTER IS TO EXPRESS INFORMATION/F.

No. 14. EXISTENCE.

INFORMATION/F IS MANIFESTED BY MOTION IN E/MATTER; ALL E/MATTER HAS MOTION, THEREFORE ALL E/MATTER HAS EXISTENCE.

No.15. NO MOTION WITHOUT INSTRUCTIVE INFORMATION/F.

E/MATTER CAN HAVE NO MOTION WITHOUT INSTRUCTIVE INFORMATION/F ORGANIZED BY THE PRINCIPLE OF ORGANIZATION.

No. 16. ORGANIZATION IN BOTH INORGANIC AND ORGANIC E/MATTER.

A UNIVERSAL PRINCIPLE OF ORGANIZATION ORGANIZES INFORMATION/F OF BOTH ORGANIC AND INORGANIC E/MATTER.

No. 17. CAUSE AND EFFECT.

EVERY EFFECT HAS A CAUSE AND EVERY CAUSE HAS EFFECTS.

No. 18. EVIDENCE OF LIFE.

THE SIGNS OF LIFE ARE EVIDENCE OF THE ADAPTIVE ORGANIZATION OF LIFE.

No. 19. ORGANIC E/MATTER.

THE MATERIAL OF THE BODY OF A LIVING THING IS ORGANIC E/MATTER.

No. 20. INNATE LAW OF LIVNG THINGS.

A LIVING THING HAS AN INBORN ORGANIZING PRINCIPLE GOVERNING ITS BODY, CALLED THE INNATE LAW OF LIVING THINGS.

No. 21. THE PURPOSE OF THE INNATE LAW OF LIVING THINGS.

THE PURPOSE OF THE INNATE LAW OF LIVING THINGS IS TO MAINTAIN THE MATERIAL OF THE BODY OF A LIVING THING ALIVE.

No. 22. THE QUALITY OF THE INNATE LAW OF LIVING THINGS.

THE INNATE LAW OF LIVING THINGS IS ALWAYS 100%/PERFECT FOR ALL LIVING E/MATTER.

No. 23. THE FUNCTION OF THE INNATE LAW OF LIVING THINGS.

THE FUNCTION OF THE INNATE LAW OF LIVING THINGS IS TO ADAPT UNIVERSAL INFORMATION/F AND E/MATTER FOR USE IN THE BODY, SO THAT ALL PARTS OF THE BODY WILL HAVE COORDINATED ACTION FOR MUTUAL BENEFIT.

No. 24. THE LIMITS OF ADAPTATION.

THE INNATE LAW OF LIVING THINGS ADAPTS INFORMATION/F AND E/MATTER FOR THE BODY ONLY IF IT IS POSSIBLE ACCORDING TO UNIVERSAL LAWS.

No. 25. THE CHARACTER OF INNATE INFORMATION/F.

THE INFORMATION/F OF THE INNATE LAW OF LIVING THINGS NEVER INJURES OR DE-CONSTRUCTS THE STRUCTURES IN WHICH IT WORKS.

No. 26. COMPARISON OF UNIVERSAL INFORMATION/F AND INNATE INFORMATION/F.

IN ORDER TO CARRY ON THE UNIVERSAL CYCLE OF LIFE, UNIVERSAL INFORMATION/F IS DE-CONSTRUCTIVE, AND INNATE INFORMATION/F IS RE-CONSTRUCTIVE, AS REGARDS TO STRUCTURAL E/MATTER.

No. 27. THE NORMALITY OF THE INNATE LAW OF LIVING THINGS.

THE INNATE LAW OF LIVING THINGS IS ALWAYS NORMAL AND ITS FUNCTION IS ALWAYS NORMAL.

No. 28. THE CONDUCTORS OF INNATE INFORMATION/F.

THE CONDUCTED INFORMATION/F OF THE INNATE LAW OF LIVING THINGS OPERATES THROUGH OR OVER THE NERVOUS SYSTEM IN ANIMAL BODIES.

No. 29. INTERFERENCE WITH TRANSMISSION OF CONDUCTED INNATE INFORMATION/F.

THERE CAN BE INTERFERENCE WITH THE TRANSMISSION OF CONDUCTED INNATE INFORMATION/F.

No. 30. THE CAUSES OF DIS-EASE.

INTERFERENCE WITH TRANSMISSION OF CONDUCTED INNATE INFORMATION/F CAUSES INCOORDINATION OF DIS-EASE.

No. 31. VERTEBRAL SUBLUXATIONS.

INTERFERENCE WITH CONDUCTED INNATE INFORMATION/F IS ALWAYS DIRECTLY OR INDIRECTLY DUE TO VERTEBRAL SUBLUXATIONS.

No. 32. THE PRINCIPLE OF COORDINATION.

COORDINATION IS THE PRINCIPLE OF COHERENT ACTIONS OF ALL THE PARTS OF AN ORGANISM IN FULFILLING THEIR ROLES AND PURPOSES.

No. 33. THE PRINCIPLE OF CONTINUOUS SUPPLY AND COMPUTATION.

THE PRINCIPLE OF CONTINUOUS SUPPLY AND COMPUTATION IS EXISTENT IN THE BODY IN ITS IDEAL STATE; WHEREIN THE LIVING BODY IS THE "COMPUTER," THE INNATE LAW IS THE "NORMAL SOFTWARE," THE INNATE FIELD IS THE "OPERATING SYSTEM," THE PHYSICAL BRAIN IS THE "CENTRAL PROCESSING UNIT," THE BRAIN CELLS ARE THE "PROCESSORS," AND THE NERVE CELLS ARE THE "TRANSMITTERS."

TURNING CHIROPRACTIC ON ITS HEAD

Stephenson wrote, "The story that is the explanation of the cyclic steps may be reversed; that is, going from the effect to the cause and from the cause back to the effect. The place to start reasoning is always at the cause or at the effect."[1: p.67]

Let us describe the narrative from principle #33 all the way up to principle #1. It is an explanation of chiropractic that is **hard to vary**, that is bidirectional, and it has **universal** value. Let us see, without condemnation, if it is true. If it is true, then let us consider reconstructing the chiropractic orientation for now as we apply the principle of continuous supply and computation (pri. 33) as the analogy; this will provide NEW educational knowledge, for the public, toward a greater understanding of chiropractic over the next 5000 years. After all, chiropractic is a humanitarian evolutionary approach to life.[17]

The nervous system is the medium used to transmit innate impulses in vertebrate animal bodies (pri. 28). Of course, even though human beings belong to the animal kingdom, we know that we are much more than animals. The law of continuous supply and computation is existent in the body (pri. 33); the body is really a universal computer governed by the innate law to maintain it **as living** (pri. 21), only if **it is possible,** within the limitations of E/matter (pri. 24). Of course, even though the human body computes informational data, like a universal computer does, we know that we are much more than computers. As we invert the process and we move from specific to general, you will notice the necessity to constantly make assumptions that are indicative of inductive reasoning. This will underscore the importance of chiropractic as a deductive science.[1: p.xvi] Throughout this process, the law of continuous supply and computation will be used along with the analogy of the universal computer. It will provide a systematic congruency that will supply the student with further insights regarding to the irrefutable veracity of chiropractic as a "radical science".[1: p.xvi]

UPSIDE-DOWN-FROM-BELOW-UP
(IN REVERSE)

Let us verify or falsify Dr. Stephenson's assertion that "the explanation of the cyclic steps may be reversed." For coordination of activities, "The law of continuous supply and computation is at work within the body of living things as per principle *#33*. The major differentiation between the operations of a sophisticated computer and those of the complex body of a living thing is the nature of its software. The software of a computer requires periodic updates, however the software of the body (the innate law of living things) is ALWAYS 100%/perfect, complete, and normal (pri. 22, 27). It NEVER needs updates. It is ALWAYS up to date moment to moment, as Stephenson wrote, "This force or message is specific for the momentary needs of a tissue cell."[1: p.265] The innate law/perfect software is ALWAYS normal and perfectly computing, encoding, adapting, and transmitting innate information/F within the limitation of E/matter (pri. 24). Therefore, note that the nerve cells/transmitters are the starting point of the transmission cycle, so as to be compliant with being **continually** at cause, as long as there is no interference due to vertebral subluxation (which is the chiropractic objective!). We observe that the location, analysis and facilitation of the correction of vertebral subluxations is an ACT that reveals the understanding of a specific knowledge: that the innate law continually computes, encodes, adapts, and transmits conducted information/F so that all parts of the body will have coordinated action, and that it also continually adapts radiated information/F and E/matter controlling its cellular components for metabolism of the cell for use in the body thus satisfying the principle of coordination *#32.*

If the principle of coordination is violated, this will produce incoherence between the activities of the parts of the body. All coordination systems depend on solutions to the concurrency control problems of negotiation, synchronization, codification, and finalization. Since chiropractic is about **what is possible** in accordance to universal laws (pri. 24), this finite limitation of E/matter is subject to errors in terms of the parts of the body lacking coherence, which will require error correction. The cause of this lack of coordination of action is principle *#31*. It is the interference with transmission of conducted information/F that is directly or indirectly due to vertebral subluxation. It is the lack of ease of the transmitter-nerve cell that is the CAUSE of the interference with the normal momentum flow of transmission of conducted innate information/F (innate impulse) in principle *#30*. It demonstrates that there can be interference with the transmitters of conducted innate information/F noted in principle *#29.*

It also reveals the conductor medium for the animal body, namely, the nervous system stated in principle *#28.* This data communication always takes place in a system that consists of an innate message source (data input), an encoder, an assembler, a control center and a transmitter. The innate law being always 100%/perfect software (pri. 22) shows that it is always normal and its function is also always normal, per principle *#27.*

Regarding structural E/matter that makes up the bodies of living things, the cycle of life is carried on through deconstruction from universal information/F and reconstruction from innate information/F, formulating principle *#26.* Since the innate law/software is always 100%/percect and normal (pri. 22, 27), the innate information/F will NEVER injure or deconstruct the structures in which they work. The innate law of living things always computes, encodes, and adapts sequences of information/F as demonstrated in principle *#25.*

One of the main components of the fundamental properties of living E/matter is the DNA. The genetic code within the DNA of any particular level of organized living E/matter contains limits regarding its ability to structurally adapt. It also expresses a natural longevity of all living E/matter according to its structural properties and actions. Therefore, the innate law/perfect software will adapt information/F and E/matter **ONLY** if it is possible according to universal laws as noted in principle *#24.* It points to the possibility that messages can be corrupted when universal information/F overcomes innate resistance causing an imbalance. The function of the innate law, as normal 100%/perfect software, is to compute, encode, and adapt information/F and E/matter; the instructive message (data input) is an innate impulse that is ALWAYS constructive and useful for the body. All parts can then interactively relate with coordinated activities through an action loop system as a foundational element, articulated in principle *#23.* This innate normal software always balances transition flows among all the complex states of organization of living E/matter. [1: p.79] Being non-discrete, the innate law/perfect software is ALWAYS 100%/perfect. It adapts information/F and E/matter of the body with an impeccably absolute quality control. Being 100%/perfect it governs with supreme precision ALL the networks of servers and processors within the body described in principle *#22* as long as it is possible according to universal laws (pri. 24). This in turn reveals the purpose of the innate law of living things, which is to maintain the material of the body **alive** within the limits of E/matter and space/time formulated as principle *#21.*

We observe that the governing of the specific parameters for the body of living things, requires adapting, and constructing structural computing systems within the body itself. Error confinement and error correction are much harder in living E/matter due to its highly complex levels of organization. These levels of complexities are organized into hierarchies from DNA, to cells, to organs, to systems and to the whole body, that allow continuous input, computation, and output. The actions of the body of a living thing are under the governance, programming control if you will, of an inborn organizing principle called, the innate law of living things. It is principle *#20.* This innate law is a 100%/perfect innate software that organizes networks of shared material entities, within the living body, and that activates operations in each other through interoperability by exchanging specific encoded message signals in order to keep it **alive.** We observe that the material of the body of a living thing is composed of carbon-based elements that the innate law/perfect software constructs into organic E/matter stated in principle *#19.* It follows that living E/matter has certain characteristic that distinguish it from non-living E/matter. We call these characteristics the signs of life; they evidence the adaptive organizational states of living E/matter through, assimilation, elimination, adaptation, growth, and reproduction which is principle *#18.* The body of a living thing is analogous to a universal computer of distributed systems. Its level of complexity requires 100%/perfect innate software that is efficient at adapting functions for coordinated actions among interacting agents, only if it is possible, according to universal laws (pri. 24). It is based on the universal cycle of life moving from construction, to deconstruction, and on to reconstruction over and over, again and again or from formation, to deformation, and on to reformation over and over, again and again. In other words, its movement is from order, to disorder, and on to reorder over and over, again and again. It demonstrates cause and effect, which is principle *#17.*

Through observation, we notice that the natural levels of organization include facets that are elemental and simple as well. As we move toward more simple levels of organization we encounter more condensed E/matter with strong bonds, that possesses properties and actions that are non-adaptive and more fundamental in their nature. This simple condensed E/matter is called inorganic E/matter noted in principle *#16.* The organization of inorganic (and organic) E/matter is governed through a universal principle using a non-discrete operating system, (analogous to the non-discrete universal computer called the "Turing Machine"), which is a computer that computes anything in the universe that can be computed. This universal principle continually **maintains** all E/matter in existence and its function is to organize all E/matter unfolding in the universe. It computes and organizes the motion of E/matter that is under the pressure of universal information/F noted in principle *#15.* This motion is manifested in all E/matter demonstrating existence stated in principle *#14.* Motion manifested by E/matter is the result of its expressing information/F, principle *#13.* One of the characteristics of information/F, as input of a non-discrete universal principle, is that this instructive information/F can compress properties and actions organizing condensed E/matter. There can be interference with the communication of these instructive messages. Universal information/F that is conveyed from a source through a medium, in the form of conduction or radiation, or oscillation to a receiver, is subject to interference. The instructive information/F from the organizing principle that is conveyed to E/matter can be interfered with, as shown in principle *#12.* There are plenty of examples of interference (umbrellas interfering with sunrays, shelters providing protection from storms, cold, heat, wind, etc...). Universal information/F is continually computed and organized; universal information/F is manifested by universal laws and have no concerns for any structures of E/matter as stated in principle *#11.* They are involved in the decaying and decomposition process of E/matter deconstructing it to its most stable and perfect level of organization, the atomic level, only to be re-used for reorganization over and over and over and again and again. The actual function of information/F, that is radiated, oscillated, or conducted is an input of instructions that becomes the interface between the physical and the non-physical, the material and the non-material, the discrete and the non-discrete governed by a universal principle of organization. This interface is actually the union of E/matter with the organizing principle manifesting motion of E/matter; it is principle *#10,* which is this **uniting** factor used by the organizing principle that **maintains** E/matter in existence through the supplying of its properties and actions from the configurations and velocities of its electrons, protons, and neutrons.

It is established that the organizing innate law of the material of living E/matter is non-discrete and 100%/perfect for every living thing (pri. 22); the innate law is an essential extension of the universal principle operating through more complex levels of organization of E/matter. B.J. Palmer wrote, "Innate Intelligence referred above is a name Chiropractors give to the equivalent of what many know as Nature, vis medicatrix naturae, *Universal Law,* Universal Intelligence" (emphasis mine).[43: p.4] It is therefore reasonable to assume that the non-discrete organizing principle of the material of non-living and condensed E/matter is also 100%/perfect. Information/F is continually and always perfectly organized and governed by the universal principle of organization; information/F is the interface of the material with the non-material. This perfect computation ALWAYS brings about 100%/perfect information/F and is principle *#9.* This reveals the function of the organizing principle, which is to compute and organize information/F into instructions; it is principle *#8.*

As previously mentiond, the organizing innate law of living E/matter is 100%/perfect for every living thing (pri. 22). This innate law is the universal organizing principle functioning through more complex levels of E/matter. It is as B.J. Palmer wrote, "Nature is innate intelligence; *innate intelligence is universal intelligence"* (emphasis mine).[44: p.6] Organization indicates order as opposed to disorder. It is, therefore, reasonable to assume that the universal organizing principle of the material of all E/matter (organic and inorganic) is also 100%/perfect, constituting principle *#7.* This universal principle uses a non-discrete UNIVERSAL operating system to compute and organize information/F (it is really a universal field). It is the information/F that unites the organizing principle and all E/matter so that E/matter be **maintained** in existence. It is represented as a set of equations balancing the transition flows among all states and levels of complexity of E/matter. $R_1+R_2 \Delta E = P$. We use for example, H^2O with the property of liquid being reorganized, with an exchange of energy into the property of vapor or the property of ice. A non-discrete UNIVERSAL operating system comprising non-discrete device drivers are programmed into a network of discrete servers by a 100%/perfect, universal principle/software; it is an efficient representation of a universal organizing principle. Remember that, "we cannot give what we do not have."

The motion of electrons, protons, neutrons, and all other subatomic particles cover distances no matter how minute or how vast. Motion has characteristic speeds of resolution with complexity that measures the time and space essential to complete the computations. Any action, process, or activity requires space and time that accounts for principle *#6.*

Action requires the existence of objective reality. This points to a permanence that is complete in the universe. Complete permanence connotes existence of the material and the non-material, discrete and non-discrete aspect of the universe. Thus far, we have recognized the perfection of organizing principles and their function. It makes possible the **maintenance** of the existence of objective reality that is comprised of an organizing principle, information/F and E/matter. This is what constitutes the **maintaining** of the universe in existence. For the permanent completeness of the universe, and for a non-discrete computing system to exist, it needs 100%/perfect organizing principle (perfect software), 100%/perfect information/F (perfect input), and 100%/perfect E/matter (perfect output) as seen in principle *#5.* The universe is complete!

It follows, through observation, that existence is a triunity having three necessary united factors, namely, the non-discrete organizing principle (100%/perfect software), the non-dicrete information/F (input), and the discrete E/matter (output) as per principle *#4*. This triunity reflects the union of the organizing principle with E/matter, shown in principle *#3* and that without this union, the **maintaining** of E/matter in existence would not be possible. Chiropractic is ALWAYS about **what is possible** ALL the time.

Chiropractic's basic science is based upon principles that are ALWAYS consistent with **what is possible** according to universal laws (pri. 24). Its principles are compliant with universal laws. Therefore, from the chiropractic point of view, the expression of the organizing principle through E/matter is the chiropractic explanation and the meaning of what makes the **maintaining** of existence possible. This organizing principle computes, process, and organizes non-discrete information/F for discrete and non-discrete organizational systems of all E/matter. Information/F, and E/matter are constructed and deconstructed in order to be reorganized and to complement all aspects of modularity. It is principle *#2.*

These observations lead to the absolute realization that there is a universal principle of organization that is intrinsic to all E/matter continually computing information/F that supplies properties and actions to **all** the E/matter of the universe, in order to **maintain** it in existence. They culminate to our initial assumption, an a priori statement. They point to the fundamental universal principle of organization that governs information/F and all states of E/matter in order to **maintain** it in existence. It doesn't end there it **begins** here. It **maintains** the universal cycle of existence. It is always the beginning of the NEW. The universal supply is CONTINUOUS. It is principle *#1.* We have just now verified the assertion that Dr. Stephenson made above is true by using a considerable amount of inductions, specifically that "the explanation of the cyclic steps may be reversed." It underscores, once again, "the importance of chiropractic as being a deductive science."[1: p.xvi] Based on a general truth (the major premise), through rational logic, we deduce a specific truth (the chiropractic objective).

Note: The correction of vertebral subluxation for the restoration in transmission of conducted innate information/F through the nerve-transmitters is the EXCLUSIVE concern of chiropractic, regardless of the outcome at the receiving body parts (receptor). You can see in diagram 7, that the chiropractor's task is to address the interference at the nerve cells. Once you have located, analyzed and facilitated the correction of vertebral subluxations, your task is completed!

Doing justice to Stephenson's assertion that, "The story that is the explanation of the cyclic steps may be reversed; that is, going from the effect to the cause and from the cause back to the effect. The place to start reasoning is always at the cause or at the effect",[1: p.67] we see that the 33 principles have been written from deductive reasoning. Deduction, in chiropractic, is the usual process of moving logically from the major premise to its rational conclusion, which is the chiropractic objective. Deduction allows us to formulate a specific truth (chiropractic objective) from a general truth (major premise).

INTEGRATING THE MISSING LINK

The differentiation of chiropractic's basic science from chiropractic philosophy and from chiropractic art through the 33 principles reveals with clarity the three aspects of chiropractic. Therefore, the integration of those aspects requires that there be a link uniting them. The function of information/F is to unite the immaterial organizing principle and the material E/matter (pri. 9). This scientific deduction stems from the fundamental universal principle of organization, which continually organizes information/F that provides all E/matter with its properties and actions to **maintain** it in existence. This supply of properties and actions is the result of instructive information/F organized by this fundamental principle (pri. 1, 8, 10, 13). Thus we see that INFORMATION/F is in truth the interface that unites the immaterial with the material. Information/F is the instruction necessary to unite the non-physical and the physical. It is this crucial point that **maintains** the whole universe in existence. Without instructive information/F there would be no possibility that the immaterial and the material could be united. As previously stated, chiropractic's basic science is based on what is possible and what is not possible according to universal laws (pri. 24). This universal instructive information/F gives rise to the periodic table of ALL discovered elements and potentially discovered future elements. It is important to understand that EVERY bit of existence is directly dependent upon universal instructive INFORMATION/F organized by a universal principle of organization to be continually **maintained.** It is for this reason that the function of the instructive information provided by the 33 principles of chiropractic's basic science is the link that *unites* chiropractic philosophy and the art of chiropractic. The instructive information of the 33 principles of chiropractic's basic science, become the **hard to vary,** explanation of "WHY" to practice "HOW" we practice. The 33 are congruent through and through. The 33 are essentially the *G*uiding *P*rinciple *S*ystem (GPS) for chiropractors to practice chiropractic and stay on course!!!

All of the chiropractic fundamentals, assumptions, methods, applications, implications, and merits overlap and require an explanation that is **UNIVERSAL** and that is **hard to vary**, as opposed to multiple explanations that are personal and that are easily varied. It is the principles of chiropractic's basic science that provide instructive guidelines for chiropractic philosophy to explain the "WHY" of its science and art.[1 p.xiv] In addition, when chiropractic philosophy explores the extensive field of study that is called chiropractic, the investigation comprises, as Stephenson wrote, "a well developed science with proven facts and plausible theories based upon those facts and precise art; all of them systematized knowledge, and a distinct field of investigation or object of study".[1: p.xiv]

To paraphrase B.J. Palmer, the mission of chiropractors is NOT to improve the basic principle --- this is impossible --- but to restore transmission of conducted information/F that is continuously supplied and computed by this organizing principle for coordination of actions of all body parts --- **which is possible** --- in every phase and attribute through the correction of subluxations.[1: p.336]

Therefore, it is NOT a matter of who is right or who is wrong as regards to personal values and beliefs systems. It is whether the 33 principles of chiropractic's basic science are true, absolute, immutable and duplicable. B.J. Palmer and R.W. Stephenson assert that they are[1: p.336] and this book concludes that they are correct! If a principle is true, it ALWAYS was true and will ALWAYS be true! Let us together, without condemnation, not cause interference to **"WHAT"** the function of the 33 principles of chiropractic's basic science is, namely, to UNITE the art of **"HOW"** to apply those principles to practice chiropractic and the philosophical explanation of **"WHY"** chiropractors are instructed to practice the chiropractic objective (locate, analyze and facilitate the correction of vertebral subluxations for a normal transmission of the conducted innate information/F of the body). It then behooves chiropractic's applied scientists to demonstrate **"HOW"** to best apply and manifest those 33 principles into the art of practice. Nothing more, nothing less, nothing else!

PHILOSOPHY AND SCIENCE

As per principle #10, the tangible function of information/F is to UNITE two separate entities. The 33 principles of chiropractic's basic science provide instructive information demonstrating the dynamics of organization, information/F and E/matter (both, living and non-living). Therefore, as we demonstrated above, the function of the instructive information provided by the 33 principles of chiropractic's basic science is to UNITE the chiropractic philosophy and the chiropractic art.

Einstein said: "It can scarcely be denied that the supreme goal of all theory is to make the irreducible basic elements as simple and as few as possible without having to surrender the adequate representation of a single datum of experience."[45: p.270] Einstein was able to formulate $E=mc^2$. How do we make the instructive information of the 33 principles of chiropractic's science as simple and as few as possible? What is our $E=mc^2$?

It boils down to **A.D.I.O.** The Above-Down-Inside-Out formula includes every basic element of chiropractic without surrendering a single datum of experience. **ABOVE** means **UNIVERSAL** principle: The perfect organizing principle. **DOWN** means **PARTICULAR** configuration of properties: Every perfect, living and non-living particle of E/matter in the universe. **INSIDE** means **INTRINSIC** velocity of action: This fundamental principle computes, encodes, and assembles the perfect universal information/F into perfect instruction. **OUT** means **SPECIALIZED** motion: This perfect instructive information/F is manifested through motion of all E/matter **maintaining** it in existence. All this takes place through the union of two separate entities (organizing principle and E/matter) from a third one (information/F) using construction, deconstruction, and reconstruction (pri. 26). This motion that gives rise to multilevel of organizations moving from dense, to complex, to living, to thinking E/matter is caused by this fundamental and universal organizing principle. This continuous forward mobility of movement eventually exhibits signs of life (pri.18) that are continually adapted by a perfect innate law (pri. 20), ONLY if it is possible without breaking a universal law (pri. 24). At each level of increasing complexity NEW features emerge that do not exist at lower levels, which are deducible from but not reducible to those lower levels. It is the law of continuous supply and computation that is flowing from **Above-Down-Inside-Out,** continually supplying and computing (pri. 33).

The innate information/F can be conducted, radiated, or oscillated in bodies of vertebrates (pri. 23). The conducted innate information/F operates through or over the nervous system in the animal body (pri. 28) and are subjected to interference in their transmission (pri. 29), directly or indirectly due to vertebral subluxations in the spinal column (pri. 31) that cause incoordination of DIS-EASE (pri. 30). The chiropractic objective is to correct subluxations in order to restore transmission of conducted innate information/F. PERIOD.

The integration of the philosophy, science and art as three separate aspects united as one, constructs a profession for the benefit of humankind. As mentioned earlier, the chiropractic objective is to locate, analyze, and facilitate the correction of vertebral subluxations for a normal transmission of conducted innate information/F of the body. PERIOD. The question for chiropractors to ask themselves is: "How do we know we remain on course in our practice?" What do we use as a UNIVERSAL baseline to check and make error corrections? How do we know we are not off into counseling, spirituality, ontology, and theism instead of chiropractic philosophy as an explanation? How do we know we are not off into symptoms relief, therapeutics, musculoskeletal problems, diagnosis, getting sick people well while using anthropomorphism as a detractor, instead of practicing the chiropractic objective? The answer is found within the instructive information of the 33 principles of chiropractic's basic science. They are our GPS (*G*uiding *P*rinciples *S*ystem) to not get lost and to help us to **continually** find our way back on track, regardless of circumstances. It is possible to slip off course. It is also possible to get back on course with our GPS. The majority of the 33 principles of chiropractic's basic science are absolute, immutable, unchangeable and duplicable. If we follow all the instructive information of the principles of our basic science and apply them, then we will remain on course and we will practice the chiropractic objective **EXCLUSIVELY,** which is the location, analysis, and facilitation of the correction of vertebral subluxations for a normal transmission of innate impulses. PERIOD. Otherwise we may slip into other areas that are NOT chiropractic and be off course. The uniqueness of chiropractic and its necessity requires a constant checking for staying on course. *(See diagram 8)*

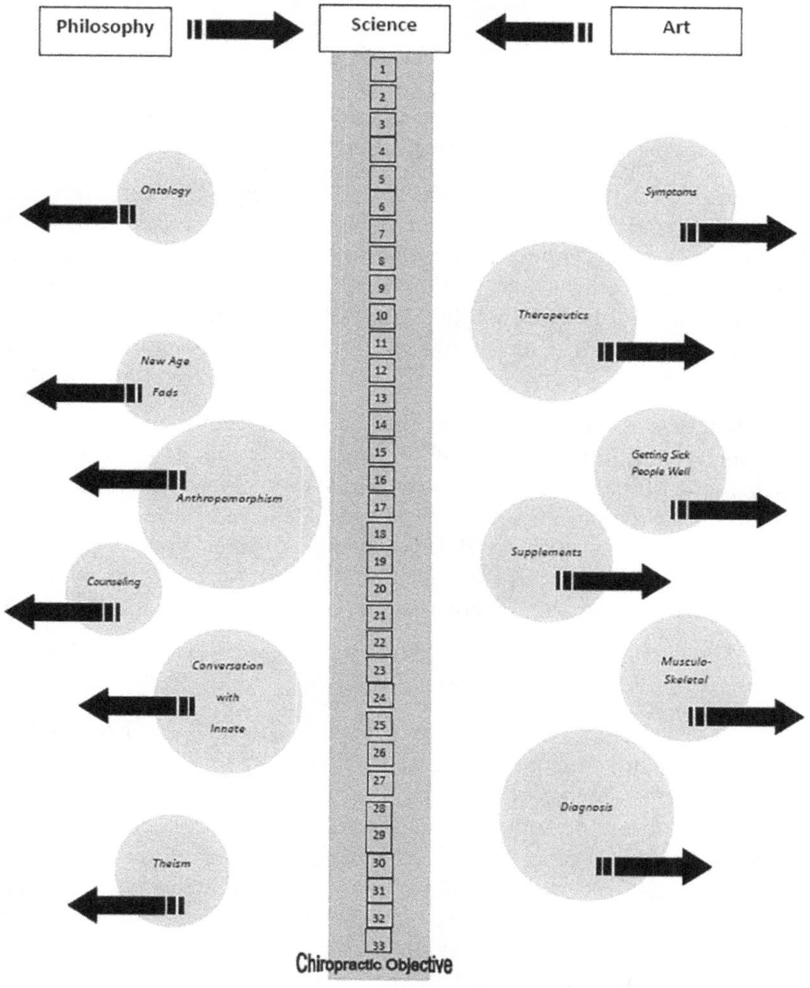

Diagram 8:
Illustration of the **G**uiding **P**rinciples **S**ystem for the practice
of the chiropractic objective. Chiropractic philosophy explains
"WHY" the, **hard to vary,** instructions of the 33 principles
chiropractic's basic science are "WHAT" must be applied in order
to know "HOW" to successfully make error corrections to stay on
course to practice the chiropractic objective **EXCLUSIVELY.**

CONCLUSION

Chiropractic's basic science has become the torchbearer of discovery in chiropractic's quest for knowledge. It can only do so by being rationally and logically explained by chiropractic philosophy and asserted by applying its principles into practice, hence uniting the two.

Chiropractic has become clannish, to put it mildly. Yet, it doesn't need to remain there. The full humanitarian value of chiropractic is based on the ever, expanding understanding that the 33 principles of chiropractic's basic science together with the growth of chiropractic knowledge give us one clear view of the chiropractic objective. Here you have chiropractic's basic science being the link between chiropractic philosophy and the art of chiropractic.

Chiropractic's basic science is the bridge that allows chiropractic philosophy and the practice of chiropractic to be congruent in the chiropractic office in order to stay on course through error correction. It is one of a most important gaps that has been identified since the discovery of chiropractic in 1895. As B.J. would say, "Check your slippings or slip your checkings." Such is the unique scientific platform on which chiropractic is now being reconstructed.

The 33 principles of chiropractic's basic science are the ubiquitous essentials of "WHAT" chiropractic consists of.

The vision is coming clearer. It is so simple that it is hard to teach. It is mostly a matter of unlearning and of learning to "see" the old with NEW eyesight. The majority of the 33 principles of chiropractic's basic science are absolute, immutable, unchanging, and have universal value for all humanity. They show us what's possible for chiropractic. It is when we unabashedly practice chiropractic for what's possible ALL THE TIME, which is its objective, instead of what's possible only sometimes, which is to get sick people well and attempting to improve functions of the body, that chiropractic will transform the world. Stephenson was clear, **"The chiropractor aims only to restore** – to bring about restoration. He adds no more current but removes the obstacles to the normal flow of that which should be supplied to the tissues from the inside."[1: p.270]

Without chiropractic's basic science, the sheer scale and significance of our deep understanding of chiropractic philosophy and the art of chiropractic, just remains a personal belief that makes sense to us with only personal value and becomes irrelevant, not something we can offer humanity. Chiropractor have been reaching only a mere 10% of the population. That's what we have been doing for 125 years. We have been flying in all kinds of directions and have we not remained on course. We have gotten lost in the clouds of therapeutics or metaphysics. All the while, our profession had a chiropractic GPS on board and we never used it. How could we? We did not even know we had a GPS on board. We did not know that we did not know! Therefore, the chiropractic profession did not follow its own basic science and did not apply it as a whole. Why? We just did not know WHAT was chiropractic's basic science, much less knowing how to apply it in practice. It went way above all our heads. We must recognize the pattern of the continuous development of our collective educated intelligence. As it was mentioned at the beginning of this book, our educated intelligence grows collectively from generation to generation as we continually make NEW discoveries. Regarding chiropractic, let us remember that it was only in 1895 that chiropractic was discovered, not before; that it was only in 1927 that the principles of chiropractic were formulated, not before; that it was only around 1970 that chiropractic was identified as being non-therapeutic, not before; that it was only in 2017 that the chiropractic principles were classified as chiropractic's basic science, not before. As time goes on, there will most likely be further updates, error corrections, and amendments that will be added to our current body of knowledge, just as we have witnessed over the last 100+ years. This is what is required to continue the chiropractic journey in moving forward and for remaining on course to best serve the world.

Today, in the 2020s, we recognize that the 33 principles of chiropractic's basic science are the fundamental instructions, with a **hard to vary** explanation, of multi level states of E/matter that is informed, organized, and **maintained** in existence; that are continually deconstructed and reconstructed into myriads of unique structures; that are continually developing into more complex structural patterns; that are eventually adapted into living things within limitations of E/matter and time. The mission of the chiropractor is to **continually** practice the chiropractic objective and to progressively understand the rules that govern the continuous development of chiropractic philosophy, science, and art. The A.D.I.O perspective will open up as chiropractic advancement is being made and will constitute future horizons for the next 5000 years and beyond.

Let me restate that chiropractic's basic science, with its instructions, is the link that **unites** chiropractic philosophy and the art of chiropractic organizing an unshakable UNIVERSAL system of living. It is a BIG IDEA and a GREAT HUMANITARIAN SERVICE. Only the future will prove it true. It will be your privilege as chiropractors to have the courage and fortitude to choose to practice EXCLUSIVELY the unadulterated chiropractic objective: then you will be **OBJECTIVE CHIROPRACTORS!**

EPILOGUE

At the beginning of this book, I made an earnest claim: I will present how the 33 principles of chiropractic's basic science are the link that **unite** chiropractic philosophy and the art of chiropractic practice; how the 33 principles of chiropractic's basic science form a Guiding Principles System (GPS) that provides the chiropractor a moment by moment situational awareness for practical correction to keep on course; how the 33 principles of chiropractic's basic science are continually revealing and pointing to the chiropractic objective; and how the 33 principles of chiropractic's basic science can move all of us beyond the confines of our personal values toward the ever expanding universal values of chiropractic itself. It is now time to review what we have discovered along the journey.

The central encouraging idea of this book is that it identifies a gap in the body of knowledge of chiropractic and restores the link that integrates the three separate and distinct aspects of chiropractic: philosophy, science and art. I call this gap, "chiropractic's basic science": it is comprised of 33 principles that provide instructions forming a solid platform, the bedrock on which chiropractic is constructed, into an evolutionary approach to life of what is possible, or impossible. As I have explained, the 33 are the "Guiding Principles System" to keep the chiropractor on course in order to practice the chiropractic objective. I mentioned several NEW points: The universal principle of organization is the fundamental initial principle of chiropractic's basic science; the innate law of living things is an essential extension of the universal principle of organization, that becomes the initial principle of chiropractic philosophy in practice (the previous principles being fundamental to explain existence); force, in chiropractic, is information; innate impulses are conducted through the nerve system to coordinate the activities of body parts, and innate rays are radiated from within the cell to control cellular components for metabolism; the living body is a system of data processing applying the law of continuous supply and computation that is existent in the body in its ideal state; the interoperability of information/F computations being an absolute for instantaneous integral innate processing; the chiropractic objective is the location, analysis, and facilitation of correction of vertebral subluxations for a normal transmission of innate impulses. PERIOD.

Today, with this NEW perspective, one notices that chiropractic's basic science is comprised of 33 principles that provide instructions to practice the chiropractic objective EXCLUSIVELY. Those principles traditionally appeared at first to be philosophical constructs, considered as mere abstractions, as ways to explain the immaterial and material components of the universe. Theism was projected onto the universal principle of organization. Anthropomorphism was reasoned and purposefully imparted to the innate law of living things. However, by considering the principles of chiropractic's basic science that enable instructive information and knowledge, one rejects this idea! That is because scientific principles allow one to express precisely the operations of entities traditionally considered as spiritual or metaphysical constructs (because these principles refer directly to the macroscopic world) such as E/matter, motion and performance. When the 33 principles instructing those entities are scientifically based, it is easy and effective to express an explanation that is **hard to vary** about the systems displaying those principles, without personal preferences. The hard to vary explanation has UNIVERSAL value rather than diverse and awkward personal values.

The rational logic of how that is done is the same for all 33 principles; it is a **uniting** characteristic. It is the mission of objective chiropractors and their journey.

As we come to the end of this book, what truly matters is whether, along the way, we have moved forward in our understanding and added this NEW knowledge to the vast body laid out by D.D., B.J., and Stephenson. As we saw when we followed the normal complete cycle, the end cycle is a NEW beginning CONTINUALLY - forever and ever, over and over and over again. In fact, the ending of this book is the starting point of NEW ones.

It was Karl Popper (Philosopher of Science, 1902-1994) who argued that, the central property of science is falsifiability. He said that scientific knowledge is provisional. In other words, it is the best that can be done at the moment. He proposed that for a theory to be considered scientific it must be able to be tested and conceivably proven false. To paraphrase Popper, it is *more important* for scientists to work at proving a theory to be false than to constantly try to prove it to be true.[46] And so, I invite every chiropractor to falsify any of the 33 principles of chiropractic's basic science as they are now reclassified. However, if the 33 CANNOT be rationally and logically disproven, then it becomes the chiropractor's privileged challenge to learn to follow its instructive information. The 33 provide the professional guidance to be applied in practice. The instructive information provided by the 33 principles of chiropractic's basic science are the necessary **uniting** bonds between chiropractic philosophy and chiropractic art. This means that if anyone has a disputation concerning the 33, let him or her take issue directly with the 33 and attempt to falsify them. The 33 are true until proven wrong. Barring this, let us no longer waste precious time with arguments based on personal feelings and preferences that become obsolete and irrelevant.

All of us together, without condemnation, must deal with the reality of the 33 principle of chiropractic's basic science, whether we like it or not, whether we want it or not, or whether we believe it or not.

CARRY ON

ACKNOWLEDGMENTS

I count as one of the greatest gifts of my life the brilliant minds of the many colleagues who, through ongoing conversations, have helped refine several concepts presented in this book.

Itself the fruit of almost 50 years of consideration, I recognize:

Reggie Gold, D.C. my mentor in chiropractic who, in our nothing short of amazing professional relationship of 40 years, never failed to challenge me to move beyond my comfort zone.

Joseph Strauss, D.C. who took me in as a brother in chiropractic in 1977 and whose dedication to the voluminous legacy of his Blue Books provided me with no shortage of perceptive insights.

James Healy, D.C. has been a consistent source of insightful feedback. His skepticism and critical thinking has helped me clarify many of the NEW thoughts and ideas in this book.

Thom Gelardi, D.C., founder of Sherman College, has become a surrogate father whose integrity and wisdom have done much to mature me.

Sara Lessard, my partner, who endures my frustrating idiosyncrasies and manages to translate my often labyrinthine thoughts into accessible vernacular.

Judy Campenale, D.C. my 'second brain' who tirelessly and generously enhances everything I write by her premiere editing skills.

Amanda Janiec, B.S., C.A., is a paradigm of organization who coordinated every facet of this project and rather miraculously kept me balanced on the narrow tight rope of ensuring that specific scientific discoveries cited in this book be confirmed by accurate verifiable references.

I am privileged to have had the support of my colleagues Bill Decken, D.C., Joe Donofrio, D.C. (Joe D), Arno Burnier, D.C., Irene Gold, D.C., David Serio, D.C., and Tom Gregory, D.C.

I particularly mean to express my gratitude to Strauss, Healey, Decken and Gelardi for the many lengthy exchanges we had that provoked critiques and challenges that served to refine and define the core message of this work.

Lastly, I am indebted to Sara for sharing this ONE continuous, lifetime of conversation and for making of our earthly pilgrimage an expression of beauty and love.

CHIROPRACTIC LEXICON

In order to continue our exploration of looking at the OLD central core process of chiropractic in a NEW way, we must be on the same page. As we move forward our educated intelligence grows and it requires that, together without condemnation, we agree on terms. I have compiled, with the help of Joe Strauss, D.C., a glossary of terms, (many of which are from Stephenson's text), for use in this book. I have also added some NEW terms that I believe are uniquely needed for practicing the chiropractic objective exclusively.

GLOSSARY (CHIROPRACTIC'S UNIQUE LEXICON)

Adaptability (sign of life): The intrinsic ability that a living organism possesses of acting on all information/F, which comes to it, whether innate or universal.

Adaptation: The movement of a living organism or any of its parts; or the structural change in that organism, to use or to circumvent environmental information/F. Adaptation is a continuous process — **continually** varying, it is never constant and unvarying, as are other universal laws. Adaptation is a universal principle — the only one of its kind. It is the principle of change, and the changes are always according to law, which is 100%/ perfect instantaneous integral adaptation.

Adjustic thrust: An adjustic thrust is a specific external educated information/F introduced at the site of a subluxated vertebra with the further intent that the innate law of living things (ILLT) will perform a vertebral adjustment.

Afferent nerve: The transmitting nerve of trophic impulses from receptor tissue cell to central processing brain cell. It is the route of internal impressions of feedback information/F from tissue cell to brain cell for coordination of actions.

Assimilation (sign of life): The power of assimilation is the ability of a living organism to take into its body food materials selectively, and make them a part of itself according to a systemic program designed by a universal intelligence.

Characterization: The construction of specific codes by the universal principle of organization (UPO) organizing universal information/F in order to maintain E/matter in existence; it is also the reconstruction (modified for living E/matter) of specific codes by the innate law of living things (ILLT) adapting universal information/F into innate information/F.

Chiropractic Meaning of Existence: It is the chiropractic meaning of all that is. It is the expression of the UPO through all E/matter.

Coding: Specific characters assignment that identify a specific communication system that is programmed to construct a message.

Computation: The operation of a computing system. It is the processing of data of a computing system using a software program.

Counterfactuals: They are facts not about what is "actual" but about what it possible or not possible. For example, Dead Sea scrolls exist somewhere "hidden" on our planet. That is a physical property of those scrolls since they do exist. That it *could be possible* to read the words on those scroll is a counterfactual property regardless of whether those scrolls would ever be discovered. And yet that those words *could be* read would still be true.

De-coding: To convert a coded message into intelligible language that can be understood.

Disease and DIS-EASE: Disease is a term used by physicians for sickness. To them it is an entity and is worthy of a name, hence diagnosis. DIS-EASE is a chiropractic term meaning not having ease; or lack of ease. It is lack of entity. It is a condition of E/matter when it does not have the property of ease. Ease is the entity, and DIS-EASE the lack of it.

E/matter: This term means energy-matter. Since $E=mc^2$, energy and matter are interchangeable; energy is simply a different configuration (properties) of electrons, protons and neutrons with varying velocities (activities). Ex: water has 2 molecules of hydrogen and 1 molecule of oxygen, whether it is in a fluid state, ice state, or vapor state. It is dependent upon the movement of its basic elements. It is a term reminding us that energy and matter are interchangeable as per $E=mc^2$; or that matter is comprised of electrons, protons, and neutrons configured with a velocity of less than the square of the speed of light.

Educated brain: That part of the brain used by innate law of living things (ILLT), as an organ, for reason, memory, education, and the so-called voluntary functions.

Educated control: Educated control is the activity of innate law of living things (ILLT) in the educated brain as an organ. The output of this activity is educated impulses; such as, thoughts, reasoning, will, memory, etc. The innate law of living things (ILLT) controls the functions of the "voluntary" systems via the educated brain. Educated impulses are tinctured innate impulses that are mostly for adaptation to things external to the body.

Educated impulse: The innate in formation/F through the educated brain, where it becomes "tinctured" or "modified" with whatever quality the educated mind can give it for the so called voluntary functions of the body. Note that educated brain "controls" nothing, except that the innate information/F pass through it. Adaptation of information/F is ALWAYS through coding by the innate law and is tinctured by the educated brain, so that there can be conscious action.

Educated Intelligence: The capability of the educated brain to function. It starts at 0% at birth and reaches its maximum at death (since it will develop no further).

Educated information/F (EI/F): Educated information/F are innate information/F that have been tinctured (slightly modified) by the educated mind for so-called voluntary functions. They are really educated impulses.

Efferent nerve: The transmitting nerve of innate impulses from central processing brain cell to receptor tissue cell. It is the route of conducted innate information/F from brain cell to tissue cell for coordination of actions.

Energy: Electrons, protons, and neutrons configured at the square of the speed of light ($E=mc^2$).

Existence: The continuous motion of elemental particles of E/matter.

External educated information/F (EEI/F): An external education information/F (EEI/F) is an innate information/F (II/F) that has been voluntarily tinctured with a new educated character for so called voluntary action with a definite purpose. Ex: An adjustic thrust.

Flow: The action of something moving along in a steady continuous stream; or the smooth continuous movement of information from one place to another.

Flowchart: A flowchart is a diagram that shows step by step the progression of the sequence operations through a system program.

Growth (sign of life): The power of growth is the ability of a living organism to expand according to intelligent programming to mature in size, and is dependent upon the power of assimilation.

Hard to vary explanation: A hard to vary explanation, in chiropractic, is an explanation that provides specific details about the principles of its basic science that fit together so tightly that it is impossible to change any detail without affecting its whole.

Impression: It is the information/F, coded by the innate law, as trophic impulses, based on the complexity of the tissue cell, concerning its soundness and function.

Information/F (I/F): Computed and coded instructions to configure electrons, protons, neutrons, and their velocities.

Innate field: a) That aspect of the body used by the innate law of living things (ILLT), acting as an operating system, in which to adapt universal information/F and assemble them. b) That facet of a living organism controlled by the innate law of living things (ILLT), acting as an operating system, in which to assemble innate impulses, innate rays or innate waves. It's location is wherever the innate law is, which is everywhere in the body of living things. It was formerly called the innate brain.

Innate impulse (II): A unit of information/F for a specific body part, for a specific function, for coordination of activities. A specific instruction given to a body part, for coordination of activities, for the present moment.

Innate information/F (II/F): Innate information/F are universal information/F adapted by the innate law of living things and codified for use in the body. They are assembled for dynamic functional process to cause tissue cells to function, or to offer resistance to the environment. It is transmitted by nerve conduction and is called innate impulse when it impels parts of the body for coordinated action; innate information/F is also radiated from within all cells of the body for metabolism and components control; it is then called innate ray or innate wave. Chiropractic addresses the transmission of innate impulse EXCLUSIVELY. Chiropractic does NOT address the innate ray/wave, even though they are vital to the body of the living thing.

Innate law of living things (ILLT): The inborn organizing principle governing the body of a living thing through adaptation in order to **maintain** it alive, only if it is possible according to universal laws. It is the essential continuation of the universal principle of organization (UPO) that expresses itself through living E/matter keeping it alive through multiple levels of complex organization that implements design, programming, self-correction, adjustability and adaptation to internal and external effectors.

Innate control: The activity of the innate law of living things (ILLT) in the innate field. It was formerly called the innate mind.

Innate ray/wave: A unit of information/F for a specific tissue cell unit to keep it metabolically sound and alive for a specific unit of time, within limitations of E/matter.

Instantaneous integral adaptation: It is 100%/perfect cooperative processes of the innate law of living things to compute ways and means of using universal information/F and E/matter for use in the body and for coordination of activities. The interoperability of the ILLT, in the innate field, to keep ALL the complexities of the living things organized to maintain it alive, if it is possible according to universal laws.

Interoperability: A characteristic of the innate law in the innate field, the interface of which, is completely understood to work with ALL the systems of the body, at present or in the future, moment to moment in either implementation or access.

Invasive information/F: Invasive information/F are universal information/F, which act powerfully upon tissue in spite of the innate resistance of the body; or in case the resistance of the body is lowered.

E/Matter (energy/matter): Electrons, protons, and neutrons configured at less that the square of the speed of light.

Modifier: A modifier is a slight change transforming a specific code through educated control that "tincture" innate impulses to become educated impulses for voluntary actions.

Momentum: Momentum is the possession of motion. It is the active movement of E/matter within space/time.

Motor nerve: The transmitting nerve of educated impulses (tinctured innate impulses) from central processing brain cell to receptor tissue cell. It is the route of educated functions from brain cell to tissue cell for so called voluntary actions.

Objective chiropractor (OC): An objective chiropractor (OC) is a chiropractor WHO chooses to practice EXLUSIVELY the chiropractic objective and nothing else.

Penetrative information/F: Penetrative information/F is invasive information/F; it is information/F which acts powerfully assailing the body and that have effect upon tissue, in spite of the innate resistance of the body.

Physical brain: That part of the central nerve system used by the innate law of living things (ILLT), as an organ, to centralize innate impulses that will be conducted though nerves for distribution to all the parts of the body for coordination of actions. It is also the organ of adaptation including the faculties of memory, will and reason.

Poison: Poison is any substance introduced into or manufactured within the living body, which the innate law of living things (ILLT) cannot process for metabolism.

Principle: A principle is a fundamental truth that is the foundation of universal laws.

Resistive information/F (RI/F): Resistive information/F are internal innate information/F opposing invasive or penetrative information/F. They may be in many forms… as physical, chemical, or mechanical. They are not called resistive information/F unless they are of that character. They are necessary for keeping the "use in the body" in balance.

Sensory nerve: The transmitting nerve of sensory impulses from perceptible tissue cell sensor to brain cell processor. It is the route of special sense functions from external impressions detected by a tissue cell sensor to the brain cell processor to adapt to the environment.

The chiropractic definition of vertebral subluxation: A vertebral subluxation is a condition of a vertebra that has lost its proper juxtaposition with the one above or the one below, or both; to an extent less than a luxation; which impinges upon a nerve and interferes with the transmission of innate impulses.

The chiropractic objective: The chiropractic objective is to locate, analyze and facilitate the correction of vertebral subluxations for the normal transmission of the innate impulses of the body. PERIOD! The chiropractic objective is derived directly from the thirty-three principles of chiropractic's basic science.

Trophic impulse: It is information/F that has been characterized by the innate law with specific modal impression of vibrations of the metabolic and coordinative state of a tissue cell as to whether it functions coordinately or not. A trophic impulse is transmitted through afferent nerves.

Universal information/F (UI/F): Universal information/F are information/F organized by the universal principle of organization (UPO), which are manifested by physical laws; they are not adapted for structural constructive purposes.

Universal principle of organization (UPO): It is the initial fundamental principle continually organizing all E/matter in order to maintain it in existence; or the initial condition of the non-discrete space/time that organizes E/matter **maintaining** it in existence.

Vertebral adjustment: A vertebral adjustment is a universal information/F adapted by the innate law of living things (ILLT) for the correction of a vertebral subluxation. A chiropractic adjustment is the application of an adjustic thrust by a chiropractor, at the specific site of a vertebral subluxation, with the further intent that the innate law (ILLT) will adapt this specific educated information/F and perform a vertebral adjustment.

Viability: Viability is the capability of E/matter to live.

Vibration: The motion of a tissue cell performing its function.

100%/perfect: A quality of being free from all flaws or defect. It is the fullness of something material or immaterial.

REFERENCES

1. Stephenson, R.W. *Chiropractic Text Book* (Vol. XIV) Davenport, IA: The Palmer School of Chiropractic (1948).

2. Palmer, Bartlett Joshua. *The Subluxation Specific- The Adjustment Specific- An Exposition of the Cause of All Disease.* (Vol. XVIII) Davenport, IA: The Palmer School of Chiropractic (1991 Reprint).

3. Dye, A Aug. *The Evolution of Chiropractic. Its Discovery and Development.* Philadelphia: Richmond Hall (1969).

4. Palmer, D.D. *The Chiropractor's Adjuster. The Science, Art, and Philosophy of Chiropractic.* Portland, OR: Portland Printing House (1910).

5. Brown, Martin P. *Overlooked!: Back on Record.* Journal of Chiropractic History. 2004 Winter; 24(2): 27-34.

6. Lessard, Claude. GSCS Annual Convention, April 2020. " A New Look at Chiropractic's Basic Science" Lecture.

7. Lessard, Claude. *A New Look at Chiropractic's Basic Science.* 2014. Self-pub.

8. Palmer, B. J. *The Value of Chiropractic* (1915) Davenport, IA: The Palmer School of Chiropractic "Chiropractic Fountain-Head". (1997 Reprint)

9. Bodanis, David. *E=mc² A Biography of the World's Most Famous Equation.* New York, NY: The Berkley Publishing Group (2000).

10. Spirkin, Alexander. *Dialectal Materialism.* Transcribed by Robert Cymbala. Progress Publisher (1984).

11. Palmer, Daniel David. *The Chiropractor: The Moral and Religious Duty of a Chiropractor.* Los Angeles, CA: Press of Beacon Light Printing Company (1914).

12. Shakib FA, and Hanna G. *An analysis of Model Protein-Coupled Electron Transfer Reactions Via the Mixed Quantum Classical Liouville Approach.* J Chem Phys. 2014 July 28; 141(4): 044122 doi: 10.1063/1.4890915

13. Strauss, Joseph B. *The Green Book Commentaries (Vol XIV-1927) The Chiropractic Textbook RW Stephenson.* Levittown, PA: Foundations for the Advancement of Chiropractic Education. (2002).

14. Densmore, Dana (ed.) *Selections from Newton's Principia*. USA: Green Cat Books an imprint of Green Lion Press. (2004).

15. Zyga, Lisa. *Quantum No-hiding Theorem Experimentally Confirmed for First Time.* PhysOrg.Com News. (03/07/2011). https:phys.org/news/2011-03-quantum-no-hiding-theorem-experimentally.html (viewed 05/19/2019)

16. Jharana, Rani, Samal, et al. *Experimental Test of the Quantum No-Hiding Theorem.* Phys Review Letters. 106, 080401 (2011). doi: 10.1103/PhysRevLett.106.080401

17. Lessard, Claude. IRAPS (International Research and Philosophy Symposium) Keynote Lecture. Sherman College. Oct 2019

18. Kent, Christopher. *Legacy and Lifestyle: Epigenics and the Potential for Chiropractic.* Dynamic Chiropractic. (Vol 31, Issue 01) January 1, 2013.

19. *Interference with Radio, TV and Cordless Telephone Signals.* fcc.gov/consumers/guides/interference-radio-tv-and-telephone-signals (viewed Jan 28, 2020)

20. McDougal, Lassewell, and Reisman. *The Intelligence Function and World Public Order.* Temple University of the Commonwealth System of Higher Education. Spring 1973. Vol. 46 No. 3

21. Palmer, B.J. *Chiropractic Philosophy, Booklet #3.* The Student Recruitment and Scholarship Committee of the B.J. Palmer Chiropractic Philosophy Research Committee, Inc. (1974)

22. Newton, Isaac. *Original Letter from Isaac Newton to Richard Bently.* Trinity College Library. Cambridge, UK. Published online Oct 2007.

23. Ashtekar, Berger, Isenber, and MacCallum (eds.). *Gravity is Geometry, after all. General Relativity and Gravitation: A Centennial Perspective.* Cambridge: Cambridge University Press. (2015) doi: 10.1017/CBO9781139583961.010

24. *Field Programmable Gate Array (FPGA).* xilinx.com/products/silicon-devices/fpga/what-is-an-fpga.html (visited Jan, 2021)

25. *The Synapse.* khanacademy.org/science/biology/humna-biology/neuron-nervous-system/a/the-synapse (visited 2021)

26. Sharpless, SK. *Susceptibility of Spinal Nerve Roots to Compressions Block.*

DHEW publication (NIH) 76-998, 1975.

27. Goodrun, JF. *Axonal Transport and Metabolism of (3H) Fructose-- And 355 Sulfate-Labeled Macromolecules in the Rat Visual System.* Brain Res. 1979 Nov. 2, 176 (2): 255-72 doi: 10.1016/0006-8993(79)90982-x.

28. Boone, William R, Dobson, Graham. *A Proposed Vertebral Subluxation Model Reflecting Traditional Concepts and Recent Advances in Health and Science.* Journal of Vertebral Subluxation   Research. Aug 1996. Vol. 1 No. 1

29. Black, Paul H. *Central Nervous System - Immune System Interactions: Psychoneuroendocrinology of Stress and Its Immune Consequences.* Antimicrob Agents Chemother. 1994 Jan; 38(1): 1-6 doi: 10.1128/AAC.38.1.1

30. Weiss, P, Jeannerod M. *Getting a Grasp on Coordination.* News Physiol. Sci. (Vol. 13) April 1998: 70-75 doi:10.1152/physiologyonline.1998.13.2.70

31. Plankar M, Brezan S, Jerman I. *The Principle of Coherence in Multi-Level Brain Information Processing.* Progress in Biophysics and Molecular Biology. Vol. 111. Issue 1, 2013.

32. Palmer, B.J. *The Bigness of the Fellow Within.* (Vol. XXII) Davenport, IA: The Palmer School of Chiropractic "Chiropractic Fountain-Head". 1949.

33. Proust, Marcel. *The Captive.* (1923) Good Press: (2021 Republish)

34. Denning, P. *Great Principles of Computing.* Communications of the ACM.(Vol. 46, Issue 11) Vob 2003 doi: 10.1145/948383.948400

35. Levet, Michael. *Theory of Computation- Lecture Notes.* August 27, 2019 p. 93 people.math.sc.edu/mlevet/lecture_notes.pdf

36. MacCormick, John. *What Can Be Computed? A Practical Guide to the Theory of Computation.* Princeton,NJ: Princeton University Press (2018).

37. Turing, Alan. *Intelligent Machinery.* National Physical Laboratory Report. (1948)

38. Searle, John R. *The Rediscovery of the Mind.* USA: MIT Press (1992)

39. Hanson, Robin. *(Thesis) In-Plant Materials Supply: Supporting the Choice Between Kitting and Continuous Supply.* Dept of Technology

Management and Economics. Chalmers University of Technology. Gothenburg, Sweden. (2012).

40. *Machine Learning: Concepts, Methodologies, Tools, and Applications.* Information Science Reference. Hershey, PA: 2012 Vol. 1

41. Turing, Alan. *On Computable Numbers, With an Application to the Entscheidungsproblem.* Proceedings of the London Mathematical Society, Nov. 12, 1936.

42. Strauss, Joseph. *Chiropractic Outside of the Box Blog- Objective Straight Chiropractic Lexicon.* April 22, 2014. josephbstrauss.com/updated-lexicon (visited 3/2022)

43. Palmer, B.J. *It is as Simples as That.* Davenport, IA: Women's Auxiliary of the International Chiropractors Association. 4th Edition (1972 Reprint).

44. Palmer, B.J. *My Message Analyzed (Booklet).* Self-published, undated

45. Einstein, Albert. *On the Method of Theoretical Physics.* The Herbert Spencer Lecture, Delivered at Oxford. June 10, 1933. Mein Weltbild, Amsterdam: Quierdo Verlag, 1934.

46. Popper, Karl. *The Logic of Scientific Discovery.* (1959) London and New York: Routledge Classics (1992 Reprint).

FOREWORD REFERENCES

Stephenson RW: Chiropractic Textbook. Palmer School of Chiropractic. Davenport, IA. 1927. 1948 Edition.

The History of Quantum Physics. The Information Philosopher. https://www.informationphilosopher.com/quantum/history/

What is Quantum Physics? Caltech Science Exchange. https://scienceexchange.caltech.edu/topics/quantum-science-explained/quantum-physics

Quantum Physics Lady. Encyclopedia of Quantum Physics and Philosophy of Science. http://www.quantumphysicslady.org/glossary/momentum/

CURRICULUM VITAE
DR. CLAUDE LESSARD

- B.S. Limestone College, Gaffney, S.C. 1977

- Doctor Of Chiropractic Degree, Sherman College Of Straight Chiropractic (S.C.S.C), Spartanburg, S.C. 1977

- Internship, S.C.S.C. 1977

- Recipient Of The B.J. Palmer Chiropractic Philosophy Distinction Award, S.C.S.C.1977

- Diplomate Of The National Board Of Chiropractic Examiners

- Certified For Preliminary Professional Education #C35301, Commonwealth Of Pennsylvania

- Commonwealth Of Pennsylvania License #DC-1702-L

- Co-Founder And Charter Member Of ADIO Institute Of Straight Chiropractic 1978

- Student Referral Counselor, ADIO I.S.C. 1978-1981

- Assistant Professor Of Chiropractic Philosphy, Adio I.S.C. 1978-1980

- Co-Developer of The ADIO Analysis 1978

- Administrative Dean Of ADIO I.S.C. 1979-1980

- Associate Professor Of Chiropractic Technique, ADIO I.S.C. 1980-1981

- Director Community Health Center, ADIO I.S.C. 1980-1981

- Member Chiropractic Life Fellowship Of Pennsylvania

- Member Of The Federation Of Straight Chiropractors Organization (F.S.C.O.)

- Graduate Of Church Ministry Program, St. Charles Borromeo Seminary 1983-1987

- Certified Myotech Examiner

- Chiropractor Of The Month Award, Markson Management Services, 1988

- Chiropractor Of The Year Award, Markson Management Services, 1992

- Post Graduate Course Of Study In Applied Spinal Biomechanics From The Aragona Spinal Biomechanic Engineering Laboratory, Inc. 1992

- Chiropractor Of The Year Award, Quest Management Systems, 1993

- Member Of The Distinguished Board Of Regents, S.C.S.C. Since 1993

- Member Of Parker Chiropractic Resources Foundation

- Chair And Co-Author Of "Spirit Of '76", S.C.S.C. 1996

- Founder Of Clients Association For Chiropractic Education (C.A.C.E.), 1997

- Licensed Private Pilot, Single Engine Airplanes Land, 1998

- Founder Of Lessard Institute For Chiropractic Clients, 1998

- Recipient Of The Spirit Of Sherman College Of Straight Chiropractic Award, 1999

- Licensed Pilot, Instrument Airplanes, 2000

- Author Of "Chiropractic.... Amazing Isn't It?" 2003

- Chiropractor Of The Year, S.C.S.C., 2006

- Motion De Felicitations, Ville De Ste. Anne De Beaupre, Resolutions 5553-09-06., 2006

- Pulstar Examiner, 2008

- Translation Of "Chiropractic...Amazing Isn't It?" In French, 2008

- Translation Of "Chiropractic...Amazing Isn't It?" In Spanish, 2009

- Autor Del Libro ''Quiropraxia No Es Asombrosa?" 2010

- Auteur Du Livre 'La Chiropratique, Incroyable N'est-Ce Pas?" 2012

- Author Of Blue Book "A New Look At Chiropractic Basic Science" 2017

- Autor Del Lirbro Azul "Una Mirada A La Scienca Basica Quiropractica" 2019

- Keynote Speaker At Sherman College Of Chiropractic International Research And Philosphy Symposium, 2019

- Author Of "Chiropractic, Amazing Isn't It- Workbook" 2020